Natasha
Savage, MD

BREAST

Cambridge Illustrated Surgical Pathology

Breast pathology is arguably considered the most challenging and controversial area of diagnostic pathology. Many gradations of normal, precancerous, and cancerous conditions are often indistinguishable, making a clear-cut diagnosis very difficult and often a cause for intense debate. This latest book in the Cambridge Illustrated Surgical Pathology series comprehensively covers all methods utilized by pathologists to accurately diagnose diseases affecting the breast. Malignant tumors are the predominant focus, but a full spectrum of inflammatory disorders and hyperplasias is also covered in detail, and the book uniquely shows the progression of disease from incipient to advanced states. Findings are diagnosed not only through the light microscope but also through genetic, molecular, and immunologic modalities; the book additionally includes the interpretation of cytologic specimens as an important diagnostic modality in breast pathology. The book is highly illustrated, with more than 300 color photomicrographs, and accompanied by a CD-ROM of all images in downloadable format.

Thomas J. Lawton, MD, is Director of Seattle Breast Pathology Consultants, Seattle, Washington.

CAMBRIDGE ILLUSTRATED SURGICAL PATHOLOGY

SERIES EDITOR
Lawrence Weiss, MD
City of Hope National Medical Center, Duarte, California

OTHER BOOKS IN THE SERIES
Peiguo Chu, MD, and Lawrence Weiss, MD, *Modern Immunohistochemistry*
Hannes Vogel, MD, *Nervous System*
Lawrence Weiss, MD, *Lymph Nodes*

FORTHCOMING
Margaret Brandwein-Gensler, MD, *Head and Neck*
Mahendra Ranchod, MD, *Intraoperative Consultation*
Lawrence True, MD, *Prostate*

I dedicate this book to Michael and Sophie

BREAST

Cambridge Illustrated Surgical Pathology

Thomas J. Lawton

Seattle Breast Pathology Consultants, Seattle, Washington

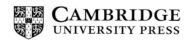

CAMBRIDGE
UNIVERSITY PRESS

CAMBRIDGE UNIVERSITY PRESS
Cambridge, New York, Melbourne, Madrid, Cape Town, Singapore, São Paulo, Delhi

Cambridge University Press
32 Avenue of the Americas, New York, NY 10013-2473, USA

www.cambridge.org
Information on this title: www.cambridge.org/9780521881593

First published 2009

Printed in the United States of America

A catalog record for this publication is available from the British Library.

Library of Congress Cataloging in Publication Data

Lawton, Thomas J.
Breast / Thomas J. Lawton.
    p. ; cm. – (Cambridge illustrated surgical pathology)
Includes bibliographical references and index.
ISBN 978-0-521-88159-3 (hardback)
1. Breast – Pathophysiology. 2. Breast – Diseases – Diagnosis. I. Title. II. Series.
[DNLM: 1. Breast Diseases. 2. Breast – pathology. WP 840 L425b 2009]

RG493.L387 2009
618.1′907–dc22   2008048748

ISBN 978-0-521-88159-3 hardback

CONTENTS

Contributors   xi

1. Normal Histology and Metaplasias   1
Anatomy and Histology   1
Metaplasias   2

2. Adenosis, Sclerosing Lesions, and Miscellaneous Benign Entities   10
Adenosis and Sclerosing Adenosis   10
Microglandular Adenosis   14
Radial Scar/Complex Sclerosing Lesions   19
Collagenous Spherulosis   22

3. Reactive and Inflammatory Lesions   25
Mastitis   25
Duct Ectasia   25
Fat Necrosis   28
Radiation Atypia   29
Diabetic Mastopathy   30
Gynecomastia   34

4. Fibroepithelial Lesions   37
Fibroadenoma   37
Juvenile Fibroadenoma   40
Phyllodes Tumor   43

5. Nipple Lesions   55
Paget's Disease of the Nipple   55
Nipple Adenoma   57
Syringomatous Adenoma   64

6. Papillary Lesions   67
General Clinical and Radiographic Features   67
Intraductal Papilloma   67
Atypical Ductal Hyperplasia and Ductal Carcinoma
        in situ Involving a Papilloma   70
Intraductal Papillary Carcinoma and Solid Papillary Carcinoma   70

Encysted/Encapsulated Papillary Carcinoma 73
Management of Papillary Lesions 75

7. Benign Stromal Lesions **81**
Pseudoangiomatous Stromal Hyperplasia 81
Hemangiomas 81
Hamartoma and Myoid Hamartoma 85
Myofibroblastoma 87
Fibromatosis 89
Granular Cell Tumor 92

8. Lobular Neoplasia (Noninvasive) **95**
Clinical Features 95
Macroscopic and Microscopic Features 96
Differential Diagnosis 108
Treatment and Prognosis 118

9. Ductal Neoplasia **122**
Ductal Hyperplasia and Atypical Ductal Hyperplasia 122
Ductal Carcinoma in situ 124
Flat Epithelial Atypia 133

10. Invasive Carcinoma, Special Types **137**
Introduction 137
Invasive Lobular Carcinoma 138
Tubular Carcinoma 146
Invasive Cribriform Carcinoma 151
Tubulolobular Carcinoma 154
Mucinous Carcinoma 155
Medullary Carcinoma 159
Invasive Papillary Carcinoma 162
Invasive Micropapillary Carcinoma 164
Secretory Carcinoma 170
Adenoid Cystic Carcinoma 172
Rare Histologic Patterns of Invasive Carcinoma 174
Invasive Carcinoma with Apocrine Features 174
Invasive Carcinomas with Clear Cell (Glycogen-Rich and
Lipid-Rich) Features 176
Invasive Carcinoma with Signet-Ring Cell Features 177
Invasive Carcinomas with Neuroendocrine Features 178

11. Invasive Carcinoma, No Special Type **185**
General Features and Histology/Grading 185
Prognostic and Predictive Factors 187
Invasive Carcinoma with Basal Phenotype 196

12. Metaplastic Carcinoma and Sarcoma   **199**

    Metaplastic Carcinoma   199

        Spindle Cell Carcinoma   199

        Squamous Cell Carcinoma   203

        Metaplastic Carcinoma with Osteochondroid Differentiation   203

    Sarcoma   205

13. Cytology of the Breast   **213**

    Clinical Indications and Limitations   213

    Terminology/Reporting   214

    Sample Preparation   214

    Fibroepithelial Lesions   216

    Papillary Lesions   219

    Proliferative Epithelial Lesions, Including Those with "Atypia"   219

    Carcinoma   225

    Metaplastic, Mesenchymal, and Spindle Cell Lesions   230

    Newer Technologies   230

        Hormone Receptor and HER-2 Studies in Breast
            Cancer Diagnostics   230

        Ductal Lavage Cytology and Nipple Fluid Analysis   234

    Use of Imprint Cytology (Touch Prep) in Intraoperative
        Consultation: Margin Assessment and Sentinel Node
        Evaluation   234

Index   241

CONTRIBUTORS

GEZA ACS, MD, PhD
Moffitt Cancer Center
Tampa, FL

KIMBERLY H. ALLISON, MD
University of Washington Medical Center
Seattle, WA

ELENA F. BRACHTEL, MD
Massachusetts General Hospital
Boston, MA

BEIYUN CHEN, MD, PhD
Mayo Clinic
Rochester, MN

THOMAS J. LAWTON, MD
Seattle Breast Pathology Consultants
Seattle, WA

CAROL REYNODS, MD
Mayo Clinic
Rochester, MN

1 NORMAL HISTOLOGY AND METAPLASIAS

Thomas J. Lawton, MD

Anatomy and Histology	1
Metaplasias	2

ANATOMY AND HISTOLOGY

The female breast is composed of a branching duct system, which begins at the nipple with the major lactiferous ducts and ends with the terminal ductal-lobular unit (TDLU). The nipple is covered by stratified squamous epithelium that focally extends into the major lactiferous ducts (Figure 1.1). Beyond that, the major lactiferous ducts in the region of the nipple are lined by a columnar or cuboidal epithelium with an underlying myoepithelial layer and surrounding basement membrane; this epithelial histology extends to the TDLU. In the nipple area, the major lactiferous ducts have a characteristic "serrated" appearance within a more dense stroma, which, when seen in biopsy specimens, can confirm the lesion biopsied is in the region of the nipple (Figure 1.2).

More distal to this, the branching duct system terminates in the TDLU (Figure 1.3). Here, numerous acini comprise a lobule, which directly connects to the terminal duct. Each acinus is surrounded by basement membrane, upon which a layer of myoepithelial cells and luminal epithelial cells lie (Figure 1.4A). Myoepithelial cells, which often have cleared cytoplasm, can be recognized on H&E alone; their presence can be confirmed by immunohistochemistry with a variety of markers, including smooth muscle myosin heavy chain, calponin, and p63, among others (Figure 1.4B). Lobular development does not occur in the normal male breast.

A variety of physiologic changes occur in the female breast during stages of development, pregnancy, and menopause. One of the more common is lactational change, which occurs in association with pregnancy. The typical histology is that of lobular expansion in which the acini become dilated and the cells within have cleared or vacuolated cytoplasm (Figure 1.5A). The nuclei can become enlarged and may have small nucleoli (Figure 1.5B). Similar changes have been reported in patients who are not or have not been pregnant; the term "pseudolactational change" or "pregnancy-like change" is warranted in these situations. With menopause and the associated decrease in estrogen, the lobules in the female breast can undergo atrophy. Typically, the number and size of lobules decrease, and often a thickening of the basement membrane is noted (Figure 1.6).

Figure 1.1. Section of nipple showing stratified squamous epithelium and densely fibrotic dermis.

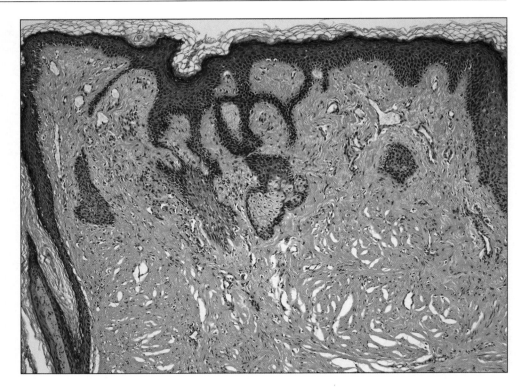

Figure 1.2. Serrated appearance of a major lactiferous duct.

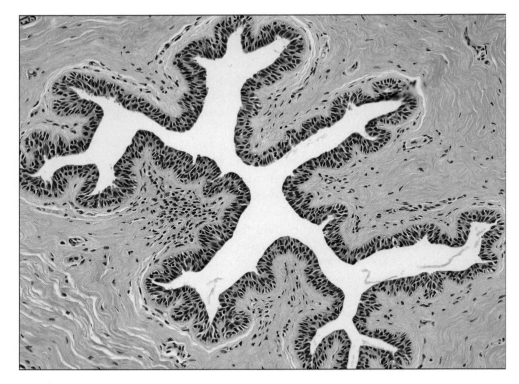

METAPLASIAS

The epithelium of the breast can undergo metaplasia, the most common type being apocrine metaplasia (Figures 1.7A,B). The cells of apocrine metaplasia have a

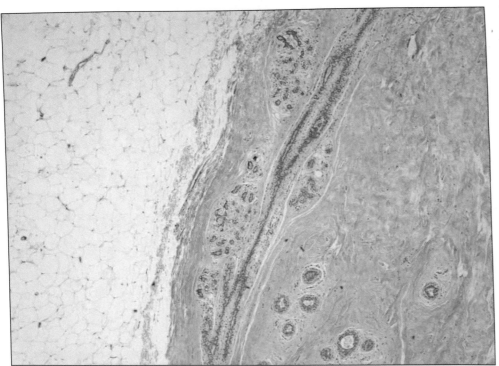

Figure 1.3. Normal breast parenchyma composed of adipose and fibroglandular tissue. The terminal ductal-lobular unit (TDLU) is present.

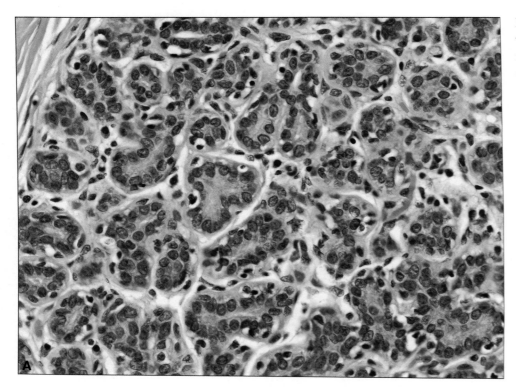

Figure 1.4. (A) High-power view of the acini present in a normal lobule. Note the dark-staining epithelium and the underlying myoepithelial cells with clear cytoplasm.

characteristic appearance with abundant eosinophilic cytoplasm and round to oval nuclei with a single prominent nucleolus. Apocrine metaplasia frequently is seen lining cysts but also can be present in more proliferative lesions, and frequently an architecture with micropapillary formation is seen. Although more complex in

Figure 1.4. *(continued)*
(B) Calponin immunostain highlighting the myoepithelial cell layer in the lobule.

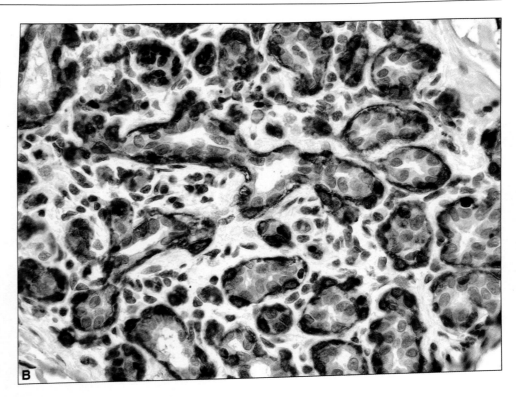

Figure 1.5.
(A) Medium-power view of lactational change with an expanded lobule composed of dilated acinar units with luminal secretions.
(B) High-power view of lactational change showing the characteristic vacuolated cytoplasm and enlarged nuclei with luminal secretion.

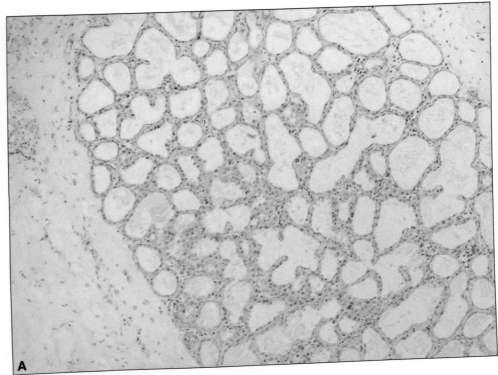

architecture, the cells maintain their uniform appearance. The diagnosis of atypia within apocrine metaplasia is a controversial one, although most authors feel that the presence of nuclear pleomorphism as well as complex architecture is required for a diagnosis of atypia and/or carcinoma in apocrine lesions (Figure 1.7C).

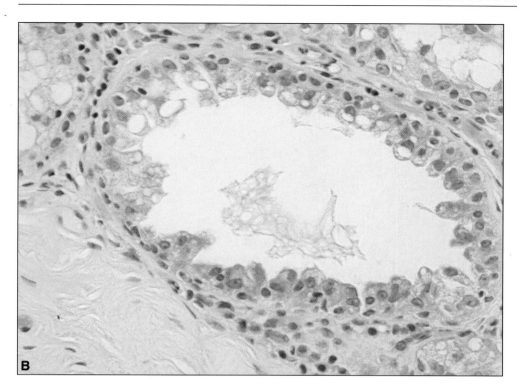

Figure 1.5. *(continued)*

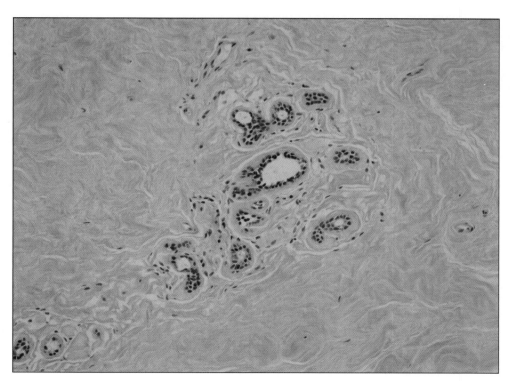

Figure 1.6. Postmenopausal breast with reduced acinar units and thickened basement membranes.

Figure 1.7. (A) Apocrine metaplasia with a micropapillary appearance. (B) Uniform cytology of apocrine metaplasia with eosinophilic cytoplasm and round to oval nuclei with single prominent nucleoli. (C) Apocrine atypia. The proliferation is growing in a more solid pattern, and there is marked nuclear pleomorphism in the lower part of the picture.

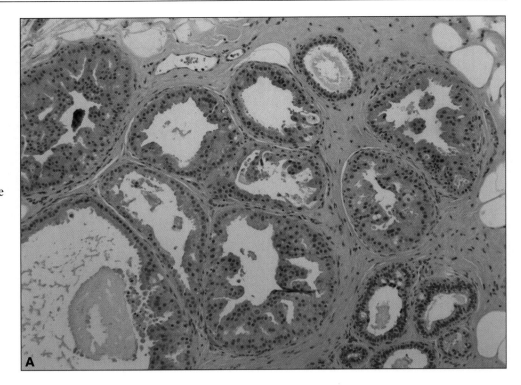

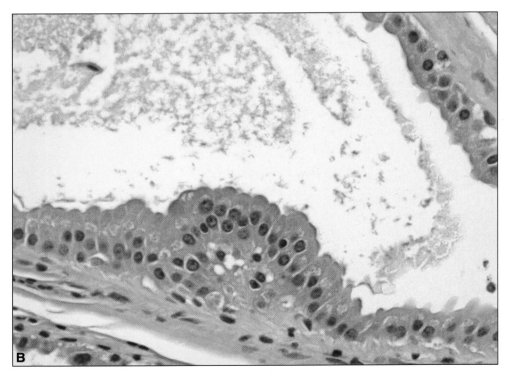

Other, less common, metaplasias involving the TDLU include clear cell metaplasia and myoid metaplasia. In clear cell metaplasia, the involved cells have abundant clear cytoplasm with small, dark, almost pyknotic-like nuclei (Figure 1.8). The most important differential is carcinoma in situ with clear

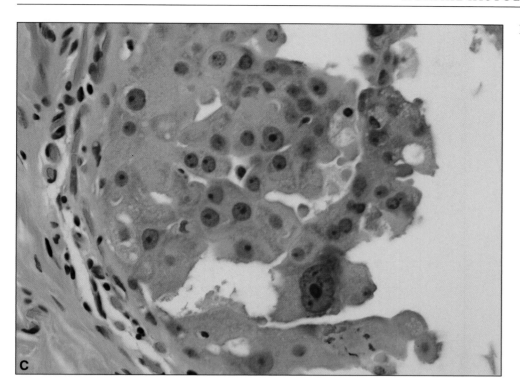

Figure 1.7. *(continued)*

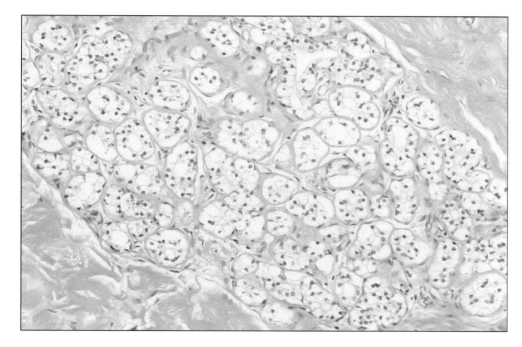

Figure 1.8. Clear cell change in a lobule. The cells have a characteristic cleared out cytoplasm and nuclei that are small and dark.

cell features involving a lobule. Generally, this is not a difficult distinction, and the absence of a clear cell in situ carcinoma elsewhere in the specimen and the bland cytology of the cells can confirm the diagnosis of clear cell metaplasia. In myoid metaplasia, the myoepithelial cells have a more pronounced

Figure 1.9. Myoid metaplasia. Note the pronounced pink myoepithelial cells with a prominent muscle-like appearance.

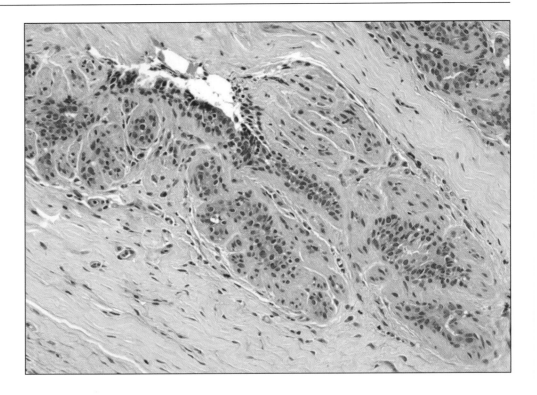

spindled appearance; their myoepithelial nature can be confirmed by immunohistochemistry (Figure 1.9).

REFERENCES

Barwick, K. W., M. Kashgarian, et al. (1982). "'Clear-cell' change within duct and lobular epithelium of the human breast." *Pathol Annu* 17(Pt. 1): 319–28.

Battersby, S. and T. J. Anderson (1989). "Histological changes in breast tissue that characterize recent pregnancy." *Histopathology* 15(4): 415–19.

Going, J. J. and T. J. Mohun (2006). "Human breast duct anatomy, the 'sick lobe' hypothesis and intraductal approaches to breast cancer." *Breast Cancer Res Treat.*

Lazard, D., X. Sastre, et al. (1993). "Expression of smooth muscle-specific proteins in myoepithelium and stromal myofibroblasts of normal and malignant human breast tissue." *Proc Natl Acad Sci USA* 90(3): 999–1003.

Love, S. M. and S. H. Barsky (2004). "Anatomy of the nipple and breast ducts revisited." *Cancer* 101(9): 1947–57.

Mills, S. E. and R. E. Fechner (1980). "Focal pregnancy-like change of the breast." *Diagn Gynecol Obstet* 2(1): 67–70.

Moffat, D. F. and J. J. Going (1996). "Three dimensional anatomy of complete duct systems in human breast: pathological and developmental implications." *J Clin Pathol* 49(1): 48–52.

O'Malley, F. P. and A. Bane (2008). "An update on apocrine lesions of the breast." *Histopathology* 52(1): 3–10.

Rusby, J. E., E. F. Brachtel, et al. (2007). "Breast duct anatomy in the human nipple: three-dimensional patterns and clinical implications." *Breast Cancer Res Treat* 106(2): 171–9.

Selim, A. G. and C. A. Wells (1999). "Immunohistochemical localisation of androgen receptor in apocrine metaplasia and apocrine adenosis of the breast: relation to oestrogen and progesterone receptors." *J Clin Pathol* 52(11): 838–41.

Seltzer, V. (1994). "The breast: embryology, development, and anatomy." *Clin Obstet Gynecol* 37(4): 879–80.

Shin, S. J. and P. P. Rosen (2000). "Pregnancy-like (pseudolactational) hyperplasia: a primary diagnosis in mammographically detected lesions of the breast and its relationship to cystic hypersecretory hyperplasia." *Am J Surg Pathol* 24(12): 1670–4.

Stirling, J. W. and J. A. Chandler (1976). "The fine structure of the normal, resting terminal ductal-lobular unit of the female breast." *Virchows Arch A Pathol Anat Histol* 372(3): 205–26.

Tavassoli, F. A. and H. J. Norris (1994). "Intraductal apocrine carcinoma: a clinicopathologic study of 37 cases." *Mod Pathol* 7(8): 813–18.

Tavassoli, F. A. and I. T. Yeh (1987). "Lactational and clear cell changes of the breast in nonlactating, nonpregnant women." *Am J Clin Pathol* 87(1): 23–9.

Viacava, P., A. G. Naccarato, et al. (1997). "Apocrine epithelium of the breast: does it result from metaplasia?" *Virchows Arch* 431(3): 205–9.

Vilanova, J. R., R. Simon, et al. (1983). "Early apocrine change in hyperplastic cystic disease." *Histopathology* 7(5): 693–8.

Vina, M. and C. A. Wells (1989). "Clear cell metaplasia of the breast: a lesion showing eccrine differentiation." *Histopathology* 15(1): 85–92.

2 ADENOSIS, SCLEROSING LESIONS, AND MISCELLANEOUS BENIGN ENTITIES

Thomas J. Lawton, MD

Adenosis and Sclerosing Adenosis	10
Microglandular Adenosis	14
Radial Scar/Complex Sclerosing Lesions	19
Collagenous Spherulosis	22

ADENOSIS AND SCLEROSING ADENOSIS

Adenosis and sclerosing adenosis are benign proliferative processes affecting the terminal ductal-lobular unit. Frequently, they are asymptomatic and found on breast imaging because of associated calcifications, but sometimes mass lesions can be formed in which the terms nodular adenosis, adenosis tumor, or tumoral adenosis are often used.

Adenosis refers to a relative increase in the number of acinar units in a lobule. Sclerosing adenosis refers to a similar process in which extensive sclerosis compresses and distorts the acinar units into angulated glands that can give the process an infiltrative appearance (Figure 2.1A). However, at low power a "lobular" circumscribed architecture is maintained. At higher power, myoepithelial cells and surrounding basement membranes can frequently be seen confirming the noninvasive nature of the process (Figure 2.1B). Often, with extensive sclerosis, it can be difficult to see the myoepithelial layer, but the immunostains for myoepithelium (e.g., p63, smooth muscle myosin heavy chain, calponin) can help confirm their presence. It is important not to overdiagnose invasive carcinoma, particularly on core needle biopsy where the edge of the lesion and the circumscribed lobular nature of the process may be difficult to visualize (Figure 2.1C). Frequently, adenosis and sclerosing adenosis form coalesced nodules that may present as a mass. In these situations, the term nodular adenosis, or adenosis tumor, can be used (Figures 2.2A–D).

Apocrine adenosis refers to apocrine metaplasia involving sclerosing adenosis. The characteristic pattern of sclerosing adenosis is present but the epithelial population is replaced by apocrine metaplastic cells (Figure 2.3A). Again, this process can be mistaken for invasive carcinoma, particularly on core needle biopsy and immunohistochemistry can be useful in difficult situations (Figures 2.3B,C).

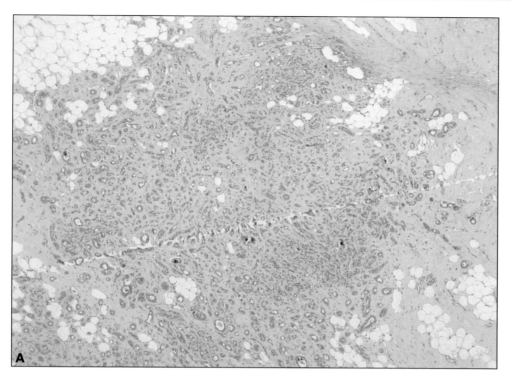

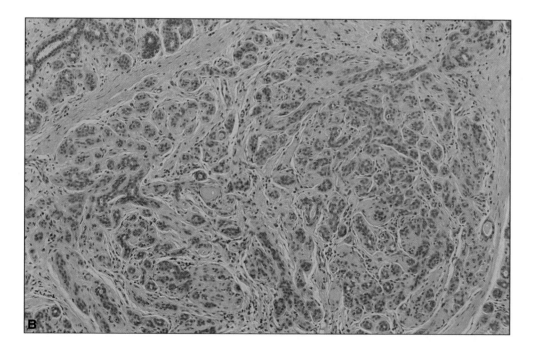

Figure 2.1. (A) Sclerosing adenosis. At low power, the circumscribed "lobular" architecture is maintained although the sclerosis distorts the glands causing an infiltrative appearance. (B) At higher power, the benign nature of sclerosing adenosis is evident by the presence of myoepithelial cells and basement membrane around the constituent glands seen by H&E.

Apocrine adenosis does not have any particular prognostic significance; however, some studies have suggested that the finding of cytologic atypia within apocrine adenosis (so-called atypical apocrine adenosis) appears to pose an increased risk for the development of invasive carcinoma, usually in older women.

Figure 2.1. *(continued)* (C) Sclerosing adenosis on core needle biopsy for calcifications. The circumscribed appearance of the process is evident, even on core needle biopsy.

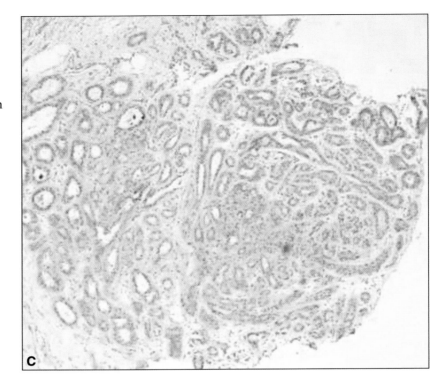

Figure 2.2. (A) Nodular adenosis. The low-power circumscribed appearance of this process confirms its benign nature. (B) At higher power, the sclerosis and distortion of the glands is evident, as is the circumscribed periphery. (C) Adenosis tumor. A proliferation of benign-appearing acinar units forming a "mass" lesion is seen by imaging.

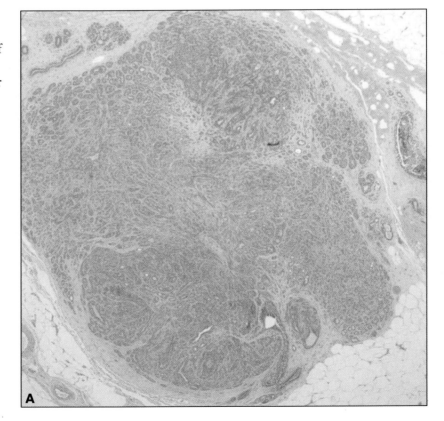

Figure 2.2. *(continued)*

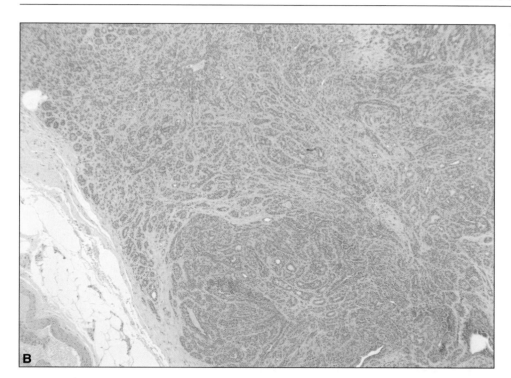

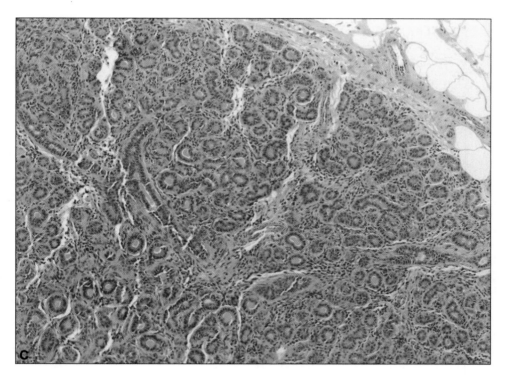

Figure 2.2. *(continued)*
(D) At high power, a clear myoepithelial cell layer is evident surrounding each acinar unit.

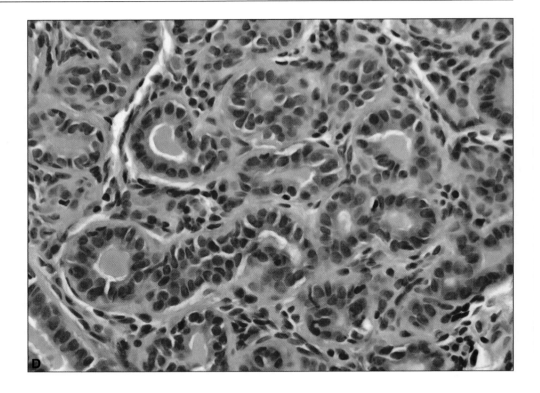

Figure 2.3. (A) Apocrine adenosis. The lesion has the histologic appearance of sclerosing adenosis, but the constituent cells have apocrine cytology without significant atypia.
(B) Apocrine adenosis on core biopsy. The circumscribed periphery of the lesion is evident by H&E even on core biopsy.
(C) However, in difficult cases, immunohistochemistry for myoepithelium (smooth muscle myosin heavy chain) can aid in confirming the noninvasive nature of this lesion.

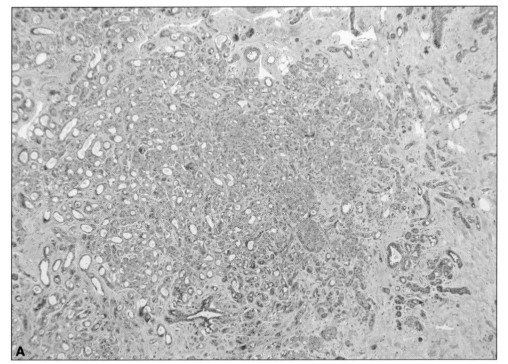

MICROGLANDULAR ADENOSIS

Microglandular adenosis is a rare tumor with an infiltrative growth pattern that can be confused with invasive carcinoma, pathologically as well as by breast imaging.

Figure 2.3. *(continued)*

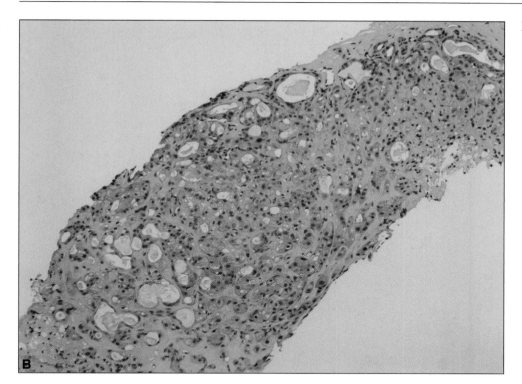

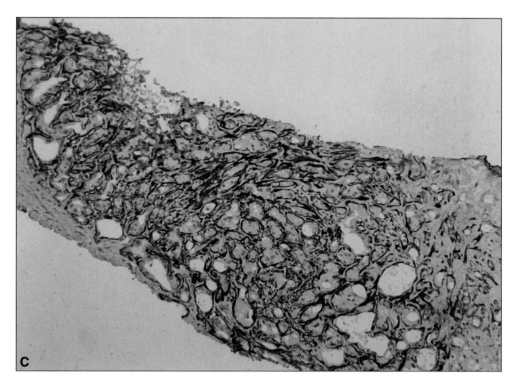

Clinically, it can present as a breast mass or can be discovered by imaging where a suspicious mass with infiltrative borders can be seen.

By light microscopy, microglandular adenosis has a characteristic infiltrative growth pattern composed of numerous small, round glands often with central

Figure 2.4.
(A,B) Microglandular adenosis. A diffusely infiltrative process composed of round glands with a single-cell layer and central lumens with eosinophilic, PAS-positive secretions.
(C) The lesion infiltrates into the surrounding adipose tissue mimicking invasive carcinoma.
(D) Microglandular adenosis. High-power view of the glands showing a single layer of cells with round nuclei, nucleoli, and an absence of myoepithelial cells. The eosinophilic secretions are evident in many of the glands.

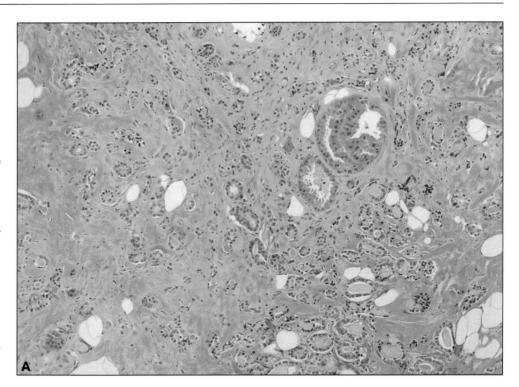

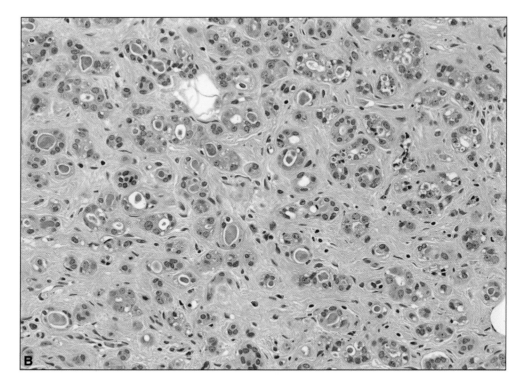

periodic acid-Schiff (PAS)-positive secretions (Figure 2.4A,B). The diffuse infiltrative nature of the lesion mimics infiltrating carcinoma as the glands can be seen permeating the adipose tissue in the breast (Figure 2.4C). The constituent cells are generally small with rounded nuclei, often with nucleoli (Figure 2.4D). They are strongly

Figure 2.4. *(continued)*

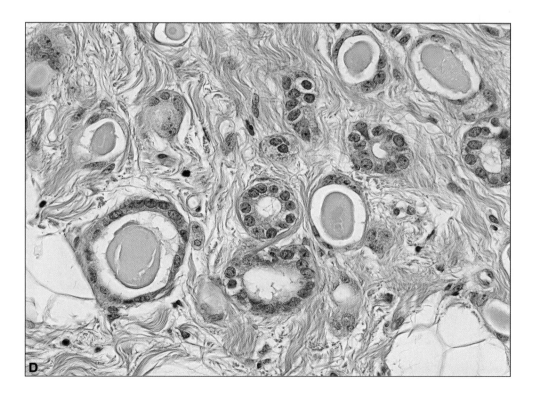

S-100-positive, and positive for keratin yet negative for epithelial membrane antigen (EMA). Myoepithelial cells are not seen by hematoxylin and eosin (H&E) staining or by immunohistochemistry, which can also lead to a misdiagnosis of invasive carcinoma. However, stains for basement membrane (e.g., Type IV collagen) are positive

Figure 2.5. (A) Radial scar/
complex sclerosing lesion.
(B) These lesions have a
characteristic stellate
appearance at low power with
a central elastotic stroma and
radiating glands at the
periphery.

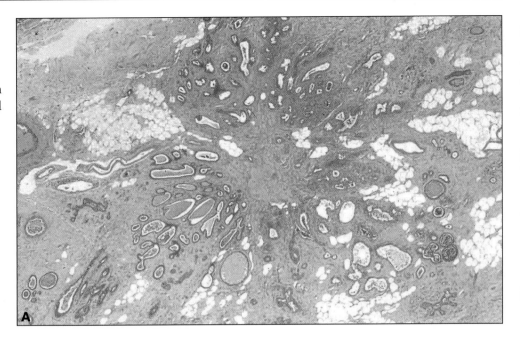

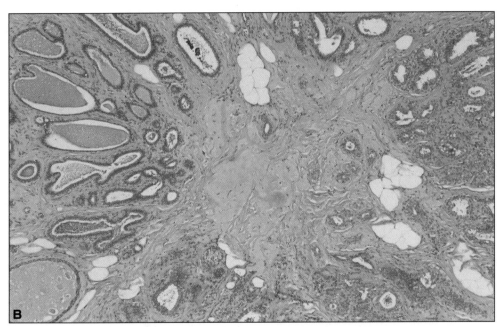

around the constituent glands. Carcinomas can arise within microglandular adenosis, and one study showed an association with adenoid cystic carcinoma.

The treatment of microglandular adenosis is complete excision with adequate margins. Due to the infiltrative nature of the process, margin adequacy can be an issue. Reports of recurrences have usually been attributed to positive surgical margins. Since this is an uncommon tumor and many long-term follow-up studies have not been done, we do not know the natural history of this process but to date it is believed to be a benign diagnosis.

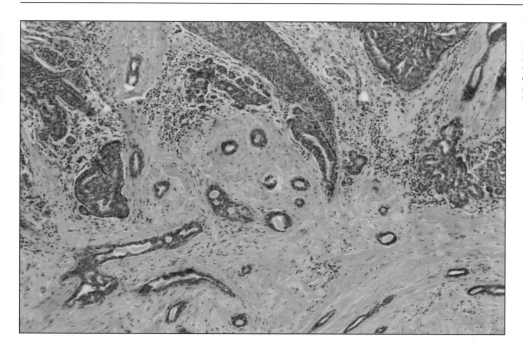

Figure 2.6. Radial scar. At the periphery of a radial scar the proliferating ducts often contain florid ductal hyperplasia.

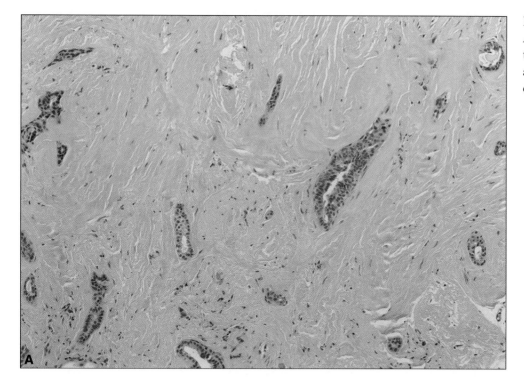

Figure 2.7. (A) Radial scar. At the center of a radial scar the entrapped glands often appear infiltrative in the elastotic stroma.

RADIAL SCAR/COMPLEX SCLEROSING LESIONS

Radial scar or complex sclerosing lesion refers to a specific histologic lesion with a characteristic low-power stellate appearance that can be confused with invasive carcinoma both pathologically and by breast imaging. Radial scars can be incidental

Figure 2.7. *(continued)* (B) However, usually a layer of flattened or clear myoepithelial cells are present confirming the absence of invasion. In difficult cases, immunohistochemistry for myoepithelium can be performed.

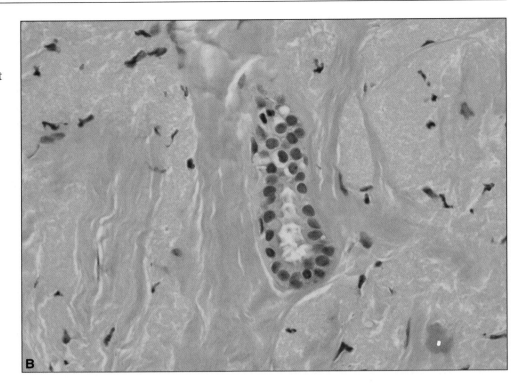

Figure 2.8. (A) Collagenous spherulosis. The involved ducts have a cribriform appearance with secondary lumens (spherules) containing fibrillar material that radiates toward the periphery of the spaces. (B) Eosinophilic, basement membranelike material lines many of the spherules. (C) Atypical lobular hyperplasia involving collagenous spherulosis.

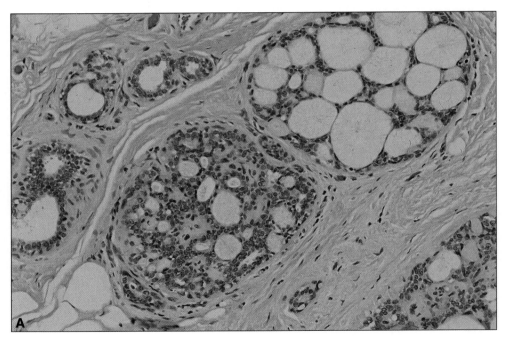

in breasts biopsied for other reasons or can be the diagnostic lesions biopsied for a suspicious mammographic finding.

The typical histology is that of a stellate lesion composed of a central "scarred" area with elastotic stroma containing angulated, entrapped glands surrounded by numerous proliferating ducts radiating from the center (Figures 2.5A,B). Often, at the periphery, the proliferating ducts will form cysts or contain areas of florid ductal

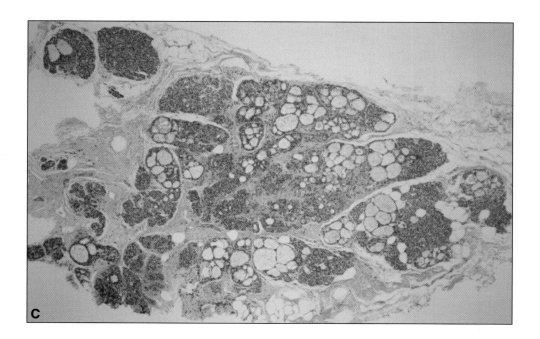

Figure 2.8. *(continued)*

hyperplasia (Figure 2.6). Atypical hyperplasia and in situ/invasive carcinoma can be present in radial scars. Toward the center of the lesion, many glands become entrapped within the elastotic stroma and appear invasive; thus tubular carcinoma is often the main differential for this diagnosis (Figures 2.7A,B). Often, myoepithelial cells can be identified by H&E but in difficult cases, immunostains for myoepithelium can be helpful to exclude invasive carcinoma.

There remains a controversy regarding the need to surgically excise radial scars without epithelial atypia diagnosed at core needle biopsy although the majority of

Figure 2.8. *(continued)*
(D) The background
architecture of collagenous
spherulosis is evident but many
of the spaces are filled with a
population of bland-appearing
lobular neoplastic cells.

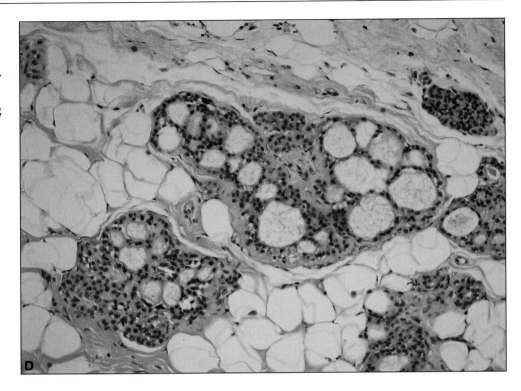

studies recommend doing so. Some studies have shown an increased risk, albeit slight, for the subsequent development of invasive carcinoma following the diagnosis of radial scar.

COLLAGENOUS SPHERULOSIS

Collagenous spherulosis is a benign finding that can histologically be confused with atypical ductal hyperplasia or low-grade ductal carcinoma in situ. It is usually discovered incidentally in association with other proliferative lesions, but can present mammographically as calcifications.

Microscopically, ducts involved by collagenous spherulosis have a low-power cribriform appearance with hyperplastic epithelial cells forming irregular secondary luminal spaces (spherules), which are lined by myoepithelial cells and typically contain a fibrillar secretion that radiates peripherally from the center of the lumens (Figure 2.8A). Often, the spaces have a peripheral eosinophilic basement membranelike material (Figure 2.8B). Atypical hyperplasia and carcinoma in situ can arise within collagenous spherulosis, frequently of lobular histology (Figures 2.8C,D).

Collagenous spherulosis is a benign finding but should be recognized and not confused with atypical ductal hyperplasia or ductal carcinoma in situ. Close attention to the architecture, lack of monotony of the cell population, and characteristic fibrillar appearance in the spherules can help in this distinction.

REFERENCES

Acs, G., J. F. Simpson, et al. (2003). "Microglandular adenosis with transition into adenoid cystic carcinoma of the breast." *Am J Surg Pathol* 27(8): 1052–60.

Andersen, J. A. and J. B. Gram (1984). "Radial scar in the female breast. A long-term follow-up study of 32 cases." *Cancer* 53(11): 2557–60.

Carter, D. J. and P. P. Rosen (1991). "Atypical apocrine metaplasia in sclerosing lesions of the breast: a study of 51 patients." *Mod Pathol* 4(1): 1–5.

Clement, P. B., R. H. Young, et al. (1987). "Collagenous spherulosis of the breast." *Am J Surg Pathol* 11(6): 411–17.

de Moraes Schenka, N. G., A. A. Schenka, et al. (2006). "p63 and CD10: reliable markers in discriminating benign sclerosing lesions from tubular carcinoma of the breast?" *Appl Immunohistochem Mol Morphol* 14(1): 71–7.

Diaz, N. M., R. W. McDivitt, et al. (1991). "Microglandular adenosis of the breast. An immunohistochemical comparison with tubular carcinoma." *Arch Pathol Lab Med* 115(6): 578–82.

Douglas-Jones, A. G., J. L. Denson, et al. (2007). "Radial scar lesions of the breast diagnosed by needle core biopsy: analysis of cases containing occult malignancy." *J Clin Pathol* 60(3): 295–8.

Eusebi, V., M. P. Foschini, et al. (1993). "Microglandular adenosis, apocrine adenosis, and tubular carcinoma of the breast. An immunohistochemical comparison." *Am J Surg Pathol* 17(2): 99–109.

Fasih, T., M. Jain, et al. (2005). "All radial scars/complex sclerosing lesions seen on breast screening mammograms should be excised." *Eur J Surg Oncol* 31(10): 1125–8.

Jacobs, T. W., C. Byrne, et al. (1999). "Radial scars in benign breast-biopsy specimens and the risk of breast cancer." *N Engl J Med* 340(6): 430–6.

O'Malley, F. P. and A. Bane (2008). "An update on apocrine lesions of the breast." *Histopathology* 52(1): 3–10.

Page, D. L. and J. F. Simpson (2001). "What is apocrine adenosis, anyway?" *Histopathology* 39(4): 433–4.

Patterson, J. A., M. Scott, et al. (2004). "Radial scar, complex sclerosing lesion and risk of breast cancer. Analysis of 175 cases in Northern Ireland." *Eur J Surg Oncol* 30(10): 1065–8.

Pavlakis, K., C. Zoubouli, et al. (2006). "Myoepithelial cell cocktail (p63+SMA) for the evaluation of sclerosing breast lesions." *Breast* 15(6): 705–12.

Resetkova, E., C. Albarracin, et al. (2006). "Collagenous spherulosis of breast: morphologic study of 59 cases and review of the literature." *Am J Surg Pathol* 30(1): 20–7.

Resetkova, E., M. Edelweiss, et al. (2008). "Management of radial sclerosing lesions of the breast diagnosed using percutaneous vacuum-assisted core needle biopsy: recommendations for excision based on seven years' of experience at a single institution." *Breast Cancer Res Treat*.

Rosen, P. P. (1983). "Microglandular adenosis. A benign lesion simulating invasive mammary carcinoma." *Am J Surg Pathol* 7(2): 137–44.

Rosenblum, M. K., R. Purrazzella, et al. (1986). "Is microglandular adenosis a precancerous disease? A study of carcinoma arising therein." *Am J Surg Pathol* 10(4): 237–45.

Sanders, M. E., D. L. Page, et al. (2006). "Interdependence of radial scar and proliferative disease with respect to invasive breast carcinoma risk in patients with benign breast biopsies." *Cancer* 106(7): 1453–61.

Seidman, J. D., M. Ashton, et al. (1996). "Atypical apocrine adenosis of the breast: a clinicopathologic study of 37 patients with 8.7-year follow-up." *Cancer* 77(12): 2529–37.

Tavassoli, F. A. and H. J. Norris (1983). "Microglandular adenosis of the breast. A clinicopathologic study of 11 cases with ultrastructural observations." *Am J Surg Pathol* 7(8): 731–7.

3 REACTIVE AND INFLAMMATORY LESIONS

Thomas J. Lawton, MD

Mastitis	25
Duct Ectasia	25
Fat Necrosis	28
Radiation Atypia	29
Diabetic Mastopathy	30
Gynecomastia	34

MASTITIS

There are a variety of types of mastitis, including acute infectious types frequently associated with lactation, others that can have a more chronic course, and some that do not as yet have specific etiologies. Acute infectious mastitis frequently presents with pain, reddening, and is usually secondary to bacteria, mainly *Staphylococcus* species. Granulomatous mastitis can be secondary to infectious etiologies as well. Other forms of mastitis, such as plasma cell mastitis and idiopathic granulomatous mastitis do not have specific infectious etiologies associated with them and the reactive process is felt to be unknown or secondary to ductal secretions.

Granulomatous lobular mastitis is a distinct entity that usually affects women in their reproductive years, often following pregnancy. Histologically, there is a diffuse inflammatory infiltrate surrounding lobules composed of histiocytes, lymphocytes, plasma cells, and eosinophils (Figure 3.1A). Often abscess formation occurs and the inflammatory infiltrate is so intense that it is difficult to discern the underlying lobular architecture in the breast (Figure 3.1B). This can cause problems for the pathologist attempting to rule out a possible underlying carcinoma and keratin immunohisto-chemistry may be necessary in difficult cases. To date, no infectious etiology has been discovered and thus the treatment for granulomatous lobular mastitis is excision followed often by steroids. Chronic, recurrent cases have been reported in the literature.

DUCT ECTASIA

Duct ectasia is a common finding that often presents with nipple discharge. The imaging findings are nonspecific but can be confused with carcinoma. There is some controversy in the literature regarding the association of duct

Figure 3.1.
(A) Granulomatous lobular mastitis. The lobular architecture has been obscured by a dense infiltrate of multinucleated giant cells, lymphocytes, and plasma cells. (B) Elsewhere in the lesion, abscess formation is noted with necrosis and abundant neutrophils.

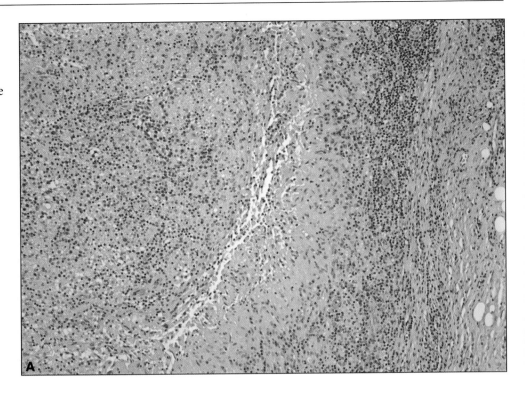

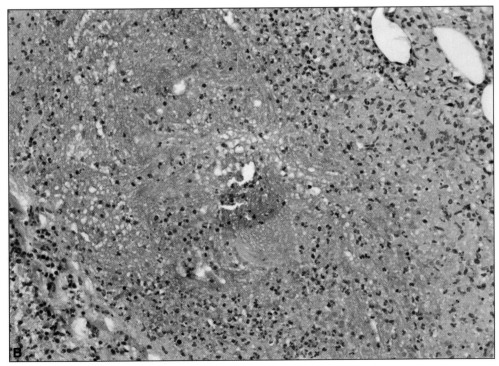

ectasia with cigarette smoking, with some researchers arguing that the association is only with periductal mastitis, which some investigators feel to be a distinct entity.

Histologically, a variety of changes can be seen in duct ectasia. Usually, the involved ducts are dilated and contain eosinophilic secretions with a flattened

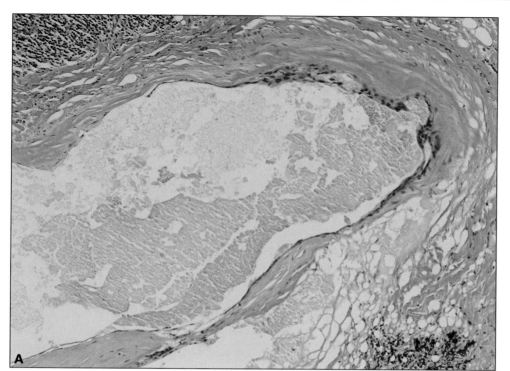

Figure 3.2. (A) Duct ectasia. A dilated duct with surrounding fibrosis and chronic inflammation. The lumen of the duct contains eosinophilic secretions and the epithelium is markedly attenuated. (B) Another dilated duct with periductal sclerosis and inflammation, and intraluminal histiocytes.

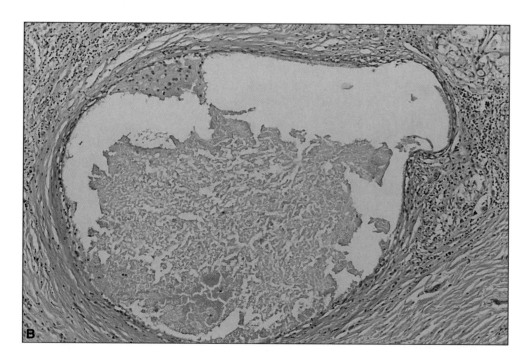

epithelium (Figure 3.2A). There is often periductal fibrosis with associated chronic inflammation. Histiocytes are common and can be present in the lumens of the dilated ducts, in the surrounding stroma, or in a pagetoid distribution within the epithelium lining the ducts (Figure 3.2B). Typically, excision of the involved area is curative.

Figure 3.3. (A) Fat necrosis. Note the marked histiocytic and chronic inflammatory infiltrate admixed within the fat. (B) High-power view of histiocytes, lymphocytes, and adipocytes. This inflammatory infiltrate can obscure an underlying carcinoma.

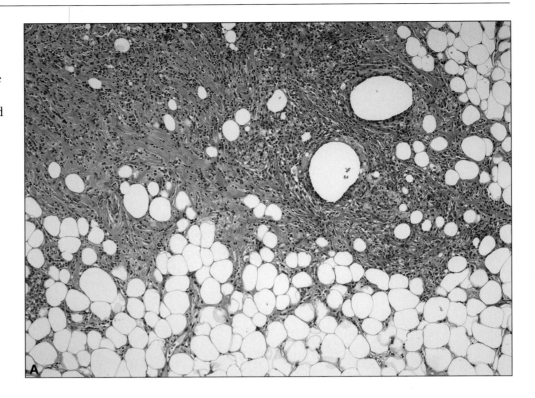

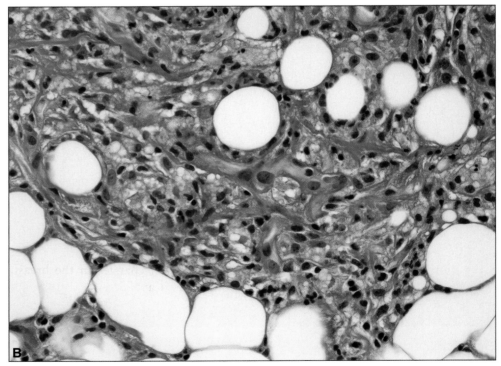

FAT NECROSIS

Fat necrosis refers to histologic findings that frequently occur after trauma or prior biopsy/surgical procedure. Mammographically, fat necrosis can present as a stellate

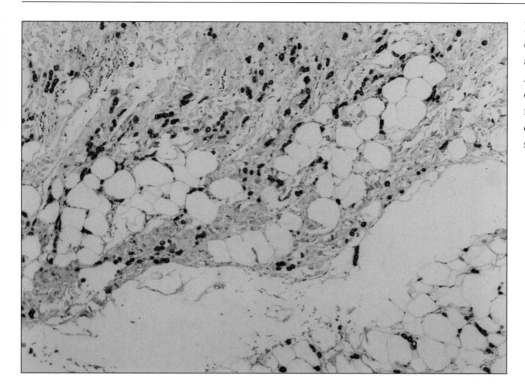

Figure 3.4. Invasive lobular carcinoma within fat necrosis associated with prior biopsy. A keratin stain was needed to confirm the presence of residual invasive lobular carcinoma in a prior biopsy site with fat necrosis.

lesion often with dystrophic calcifications and can be confused with invasive carcinoma.

Histologically, fat necrosis is composed of multinucleated histiocytes, lymphocytes, hemorrhage, or hemosiderin-laden macrophages, and varying degrees of fibrosis and calcification (Figures 3.3A,B). These changes can be seen following prior biopsies and thus can obscure a search for residual carcinoma, particularly, subtle lesions such as invasive lobular carcinoma; keratin immunohistochemistry can be helpful but should be used judiciously (Figure 3.4).

RADIATION ATYPIA

Prior radiation therapy can cause characteristic atypical changes in the breast, including stromal fibrosis with stromal cell atypia and atrophy of lobules with associated random epithelial atypia. Atrophic lobules will frequently have thickened basement membranes (Figure 3.5A) and the epithelial cells may be enlarged and hyperchromatic with vacuolated cytoplasm (Figure 3.5B). The differential includes in-situ carcinoma and care must be taken not to overdiagnose carcinoma in a patient who has received radiation therapy to the breast. Usually, the involved ducts/lobules of radiated carcinoma will not only show atypical cytology but will also retain the architecture of in-situ carcinoma.

Figure 3.5. (A) Radiation atypia. A lobule showing changes secondary to prior radiation therapy including atrophy, thickening of basement membranes, and random nuclear atypia. (B) Radiation atypia. A duct showing random nuclear atypia with cytoplasmic vacuolization in a patient with a prior history of radiation therapy to the same breast. Care should be taken not to overdiagnose carcinoma in this situation.

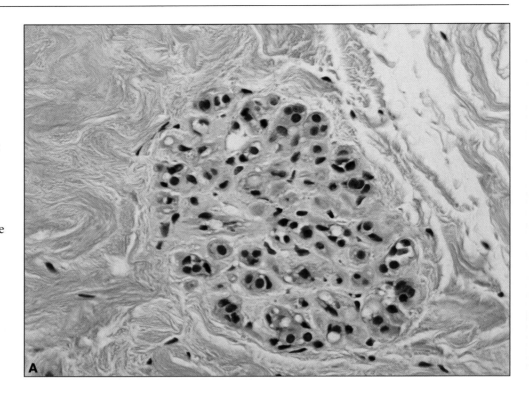

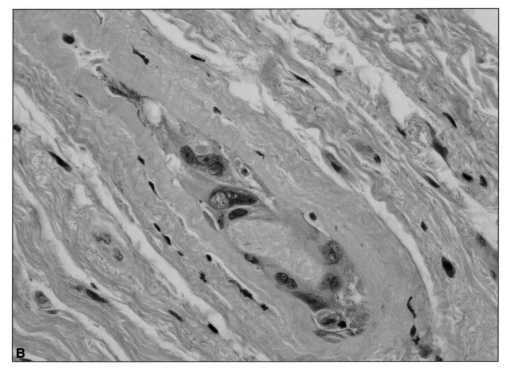

DIABETIC MASTOPATHY

The term diabetic mastopathy was originally coined to describe a distinct constellation of histologic findings in patients with type I diabetes mellitus. However,

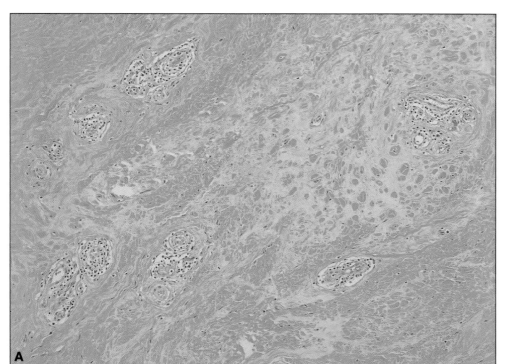

Figure 3.6. (A) Diabetic mastopathy. The stroma is markedly fibrotic with "keloidal" type fibrosis centrally. Note the perivascular and perilobular lymphocytic infiltrate. (B/C) Diabetic mastopathy. Medium- and high-power view of the epithelioid fibroblasts characteristic of diabetic mastopathy. These cells, although atypical, should not be confused with carcinoma as they are myofibroblastic in origin. In difficult cases, keratin immunostains can be of assistance.

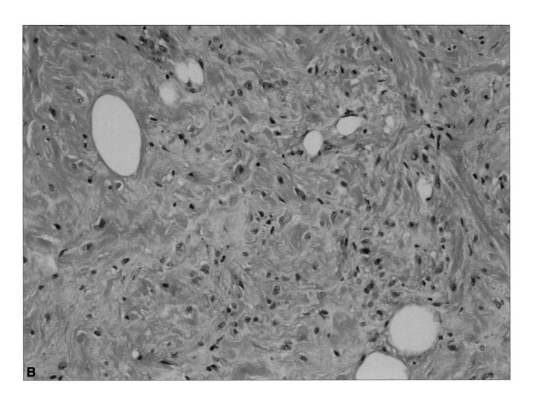

similar histologic findings have been described in patients with type II diabetes mellitus, other autoimmune disorders, and in patients with no known autoimmune disorder at the time of diagnosis. Thus, some have suggested using the terms sclerosing lymphocytic lobulitis, fibrous mastopathy, or lymphocytic mastopathy.

Figure 3.6. *(continued)*
(D) Diabetic mastopathy. The
classic perivascular and
perilobular appearance of the
lymphocytic infiltrate. The
cells are predominantly
B-cells and are polyclonal in
nature.

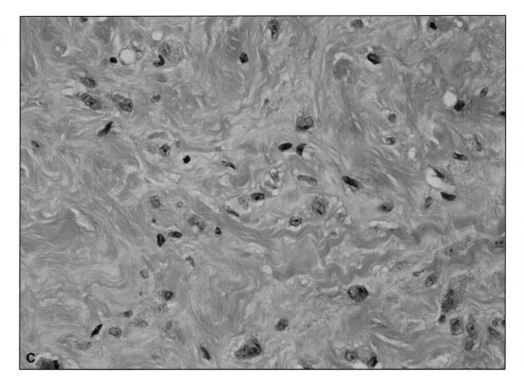

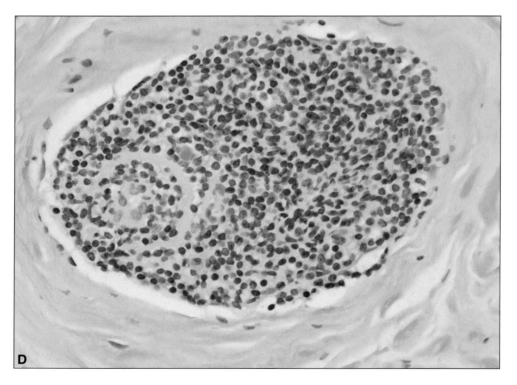

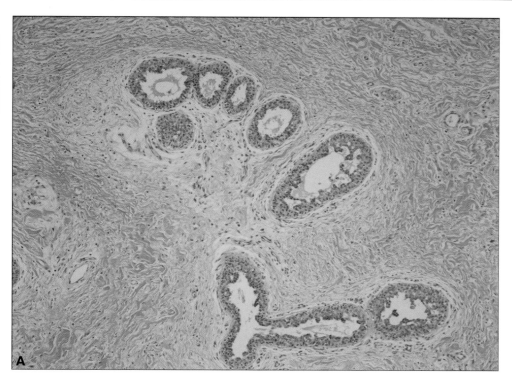

Figure 3.7. (A) Gynecomastia. The stroma is somewhat cellular and has the appearance of pseudoangiomatous stromal hyperplasia. The epithelium is hyperplastic in a micropapillary-type pattern. (B) Gynecomastia. The epithelium has a characteristic appearance with micropapillary-type projections in the lumen.

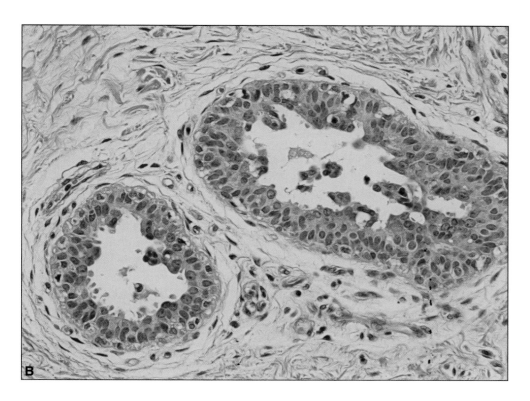

Figure 3.7. *(continued)*
(C) However, the projections taper at the center and the cell population is mixed and not monotypic as seen in micropapillary ductal carcinoma in situ.

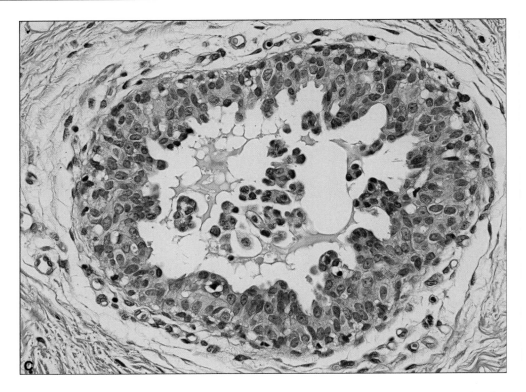

In the rest of this chapter, we will use the original term diabetic mastopathy for consistency. Clinically, diabetic mastopathy usually presents as a painless mass and has been reported in both sexes. Imaging findings usually are those of a mass lesion that can resemble fibroadenoma.

Histologically, the classic findings of diabetic mastopathy are a dense "keloidal" type of collagen, a periductal and perivascular lymphocytic infiltrate, and prominent epithelioid fibroblasts in the stroma (Figures 3.6A–D). The large epithelioid fibroblasts should not be confused with carcinoma; in difficult cases, keratin immunostaining can be helpful as these cells have been proven to be myofibroblastic in origin. The perivascular and periductal lymphocytic infiltrate is composed of a polyclonal population of B-cells with a lesser percentage of T-cells. This finding, as well as the relative circumscription of the infiltrates aids in distinguishing this entity from lymphoma, usually mucosa-associated lymphoid tissue (MALT) lymphoma. In the latter diagnosis the infiltrate is not only perivascular and perilobular but more infiltrative throughout the breast parenchyma. In difficult cases, immunohistochemistry can be used to show the polyclonal nature of the cell population in diabetic mastopathy.

If the classic findings of diabetic mastopathy are encountered on core biopsy, a definitive diagnosis can be rendered. Surgical excision is the mainstay of treatment; recurrences have been reported, but there is no evidence that diabetic mastopathy is associated with an increased risk for carcinoma or has potential for aggressive behavior.

GYNECOMASTIA

Gynecomastia is a benign finding in the male breast that can be seen in men of all ages. Numerous drugs and physiologic conditions can cause gynecomastia. Clinically, it usually presents as a mass that may be painful. Gynecomastia is frequently bilateral.

Histologically, several "stages" of gynecomastia have been described – from a proliferative phase to a fibrotic phase. There is great overlap in these phases and all can be seen in the same biopsy specimen. Typically, the stroma is loosely cellular to fibrous, and pseudoangiomatous stromal hyperplasia is a common finding (Figure 3.7A). The epithelium has a characteristic appearance with a tapered micropapillary growth pattern, but these luminal projections lack the "club-like" growth pattern and the monotypic cell population of micropapillary ductal carcinoma in situ (Figures 3.7B,C).

Gynecomastia can be treated by local excision alone. There are reports of regression of the disease following discontinuation of causative agents. There is no increased risk for the development of carcinoma.

REFERENCES

Akcan, A., H. Akyildiz, et al. (2006). "Granulomatous lobular mastitis: a complex diagnostic and therapeutic problem." *World J Surg* 30(8): 1403–9.

Bannayan, G. A. and S. I. Hajdu (1972). "Gynecomastia: clinicopathologic study of 351 cases." *Am J Clin Pathol* 57(4): 431–7.

Bilgen, I. G., E. E. Ustun, et al. (2001). "Fat necrosis of the breast: clinical, mammographic and sonographic features." *Eur J Radiol* 39(2): 92–9.

Braunstein, G. D. (2007). "Clinical practice. Gynecomastia." *N Engl J Med* 357(12): 1229–37.

Dixon, J. M., O. Ravisekar, et al. (1996). "Periductal mastitis and duct ectasia: different conditions with different aetiologies." *Br J Surg* 83(6): 820–2.

Ely, K. A., G. Tse, et al. (2000). "Diabetic mastopathy. A clinicopathologic review." *Am J Clin Pathol* 113(4): 541–5.

Erhan, Y., A. Veral, et al. (2000). "A clinicopathologic study of a rare clinical entity mimicking breast carcinoma: idiopathic granulomatous mastitis." *Breast* 9(1): 52–6.

Galea, M. H., J. F. Robertson, et al. (1989). "Granulomatous lobular mastitis." *Aust N Z J Surg* 59(7): 547–50.

Girling, A. C., A. M. Hanby, et al. (1990). "Radiation and other pathological changes in breast tissue after conservation treatment for carcinoma." *J Clin Pathol* 43(2): 152–6.

Going, J. J., T. J. Anderson, et al. (1987). "Granulomatous lobular mastitis." *J Clin Pathol* 40(5): 535–40.

Haagensen, C. D. (1951). "Mammary-duct ectasia; a disease that may simulate carcinoma." *Cancer* 4(4): 749–61.

Hunfeld, K. P. and R. Bassler (1997). "Lymphocytic mastitis and fibrosis of the breast in long-standing insulin-dependent diabetics. A histopathologic study on diabetic mastopathy and report of ten cases." *Gen Diagn Pathol* 143(1): 49–58.

Kudva, Y. C., C. Reynolds, et al. (2002). " 'Diabetic mastopathy,' or sclerosing lymphocytic lobulitis, is strongly associated with type 1 diabetes." *Diabetes Care* 25(1): 121–6.

Labit-Bouvier, C., N. Horschowski, et al. (1997). "[Lymphocytic mastitis]." *Ann Pathol* 17(2): 94–9.

Lammie, G. A., L. G. Bobrow, et al. (1991). "Sclerosing lymphocytic lobulitis of the breast – evidence for an autoimmune pathogenesis." *Histopathology* 19(1): 13–20.

Minkowitz, S., H. Hedayati, et al. (1973). "Fibrous mastopathy. A clinical histopathologic study." *Cancer* 32(4): 913–16.

Moore, G. H., J. E. Schiller, et al. (2004). "Radiation-induced histopathologic changes of the breast: the effects of time." *Am J Surg Pathol* 28(1): 47–53.

Morgan, M. C., M. G. Weaver, et al. (1995). "Diabetic mastopathy: a clinicopathologic study in palpable and nonpalpable breast lesions." *Mod Pathol* 8(4): 349–54.

Niewoehner, C. B. and A. E. Schorer (2008). "Gynaecomastia and breast cancer in men." *BMJ* 336(7646): 709–13.

Rahal, R. M., R. de Freitas-Junior, et al. (2005). "Risk factors for duct ectasia." *Breast J* 11(4): 262–5.

Schnitt, S. J., J. L. Connolly, et al. (1984). "Radiation-induced changes in the breast." *Hum Pathol* 15(6): 545–50.

Tan, P. H., L. M. Lai, et al. (2006). "Fat necrosis of the breast–a review." *Breast* 15(3): 313–18.

Thorncroft, K., L. Forsyth, et al. (2007). "The diagnosis and management of diabetic mastopathy." *Breast J* 13(6): 607–13.

Tomaszewski, J. E., J. S. Brooks, et al. (1992). "Diabetic mastopathy: a distinctive clinico-pathologic entity." *Hum Pathol* 23(7): 780–6.

Valdez, R., J. Thorson, et al. (2003). "Lymphocytic mastitis and diabetic mastopathy: a molecular, immunophenotypic, and clinicopathologic evaluation of 11 cases." *Mod Pathol* 16(3): 223–8.

Weinstein, S. P., E. F. Conant, et al. (2001). "Diabetic mastopathy in men: imaging findings in two patients." *Radiology* 219(3): 797–9.

4 FIBROEPITHELIAL LESIONS

Thomas J. Lawton, MD

Fibroadenoma	37
Juvenile Fibroadenoma	40
Phyllodes Tumor	43

FIBROADENOMA

Fibroadenoma is the most common benign tumor in the female breast. They can occur at any age, although the majority occurs in younger, premenopausal women. Those occurring in postmenopausal women are frequently hyalinized and may be associated with dystrophic calcifications. The clinical presentation is usually that of a painless mass, although some lesions are found incidentally by breast imaging. The typical imaging finding is that of a mass lesion; calcifications can be seen mammographically. Ultrasound findings are generally that of a circumscribed hypoechoic mass although some lesions have irregular borders.

Grossly, most fibroadenomas appear as solid, circumscribed mass lesions with a rubbery consistency although hyalinized fibroadenomas frequently appear more fibrotic. Microscopically, fibroadenomas are composed of an admixture of stroma and epithelium with two main patterns of growth, intracanalicular and pericanalicular. The epithelium in intracanalicular fibroadenomas becomes compressed by the nodular growth of the stroma (Figure 4.1A). Sometimes the intracanalicular growth pattern becomes more pronounced and clefts may form; however, the stroma is homogeneous without atypia or mitotic activity contrary to that seen in phyllodes tumors (Figures 4.1B,C). Often, particularly in older patients, fibroadenomas become hyalinized and are frequently associated with dystrophic calcifications (Figures 4.2A–C). Other stromal changes that occur in fibroadenomas are myxoid change (Figure 4.3) and myoid metaplasia (Figures 4.4A–C) to name a few. Scattered giant cells can also occur within the stroma of fibroadenomas and are not indicative of malignancy. The epithelium can also undergo similar changes as in ducts outside fibroadenomas, including hyperplasia, atypical hyperplasia, and carcinoma.

Figure 4.1.
(A) Intracanalicular fibroadenoma. The epithelium is compressed into slit-like spaces by the nodular stroma. The stroma is paucicellular and homogenous without mitotic activity.
(B,C). Intracanalicular fibroadenoma. Although the intracanalicular growth pattern is slightly more pronounced within a cleft-like space, the stroma is heterogeneous, there is no periglandular stromal condensation, and no stromal cellularity, atypia, or mitotic activity.

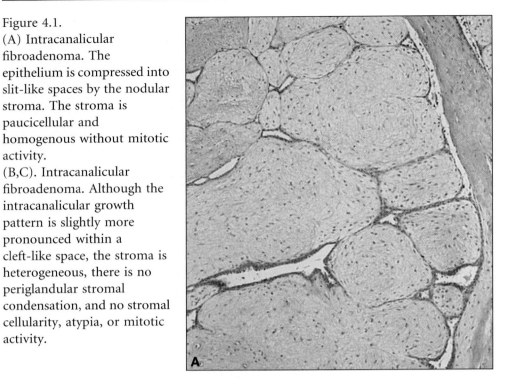

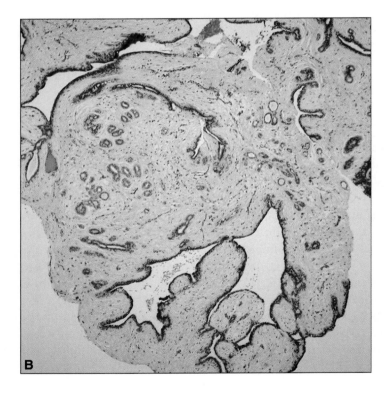

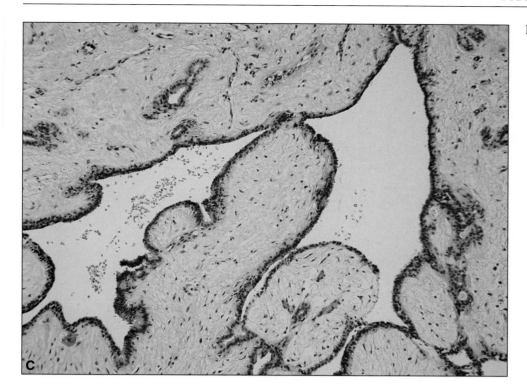

Figure 4.1. (continued)

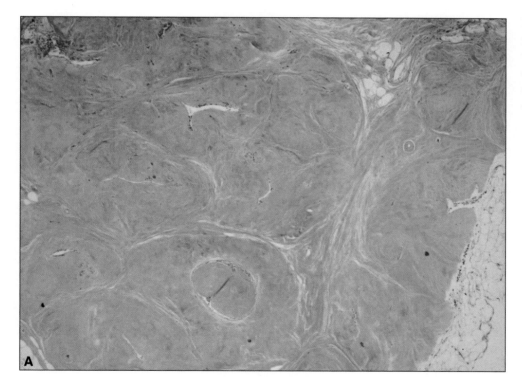

Figure 4.2. (A–C) Hyalinized fibroadenoma. The stroma in these fibroadenomas is extensively hyalinized and often can be associated with dystrophic calcifications.

Figure 4.2. *(continued)*

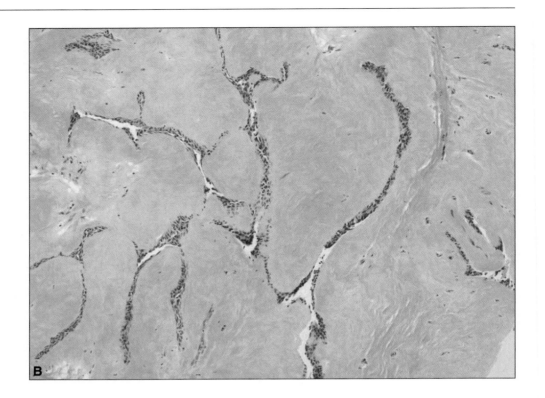

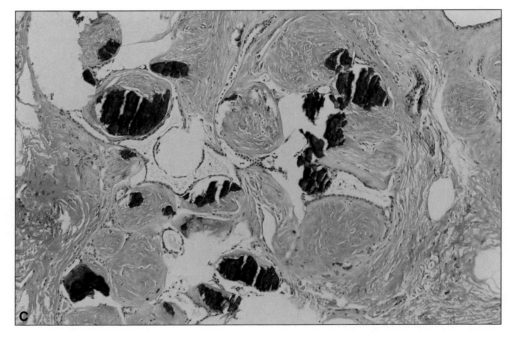

JUVENILE FIBROADENOMA

The term juvenile fibroadenoma was coined to describe fibroadenomas in teenage girls that were often rapidly growing and frequently large. They typically have a more

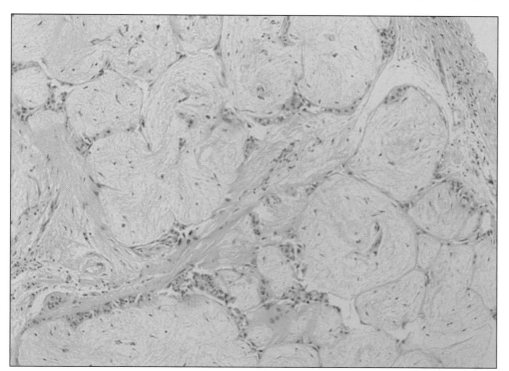

Figure 4.3. Myxoid fibroadenoma. An intracanalicular fibroadenoma with prominent myxoid change to the stroma.

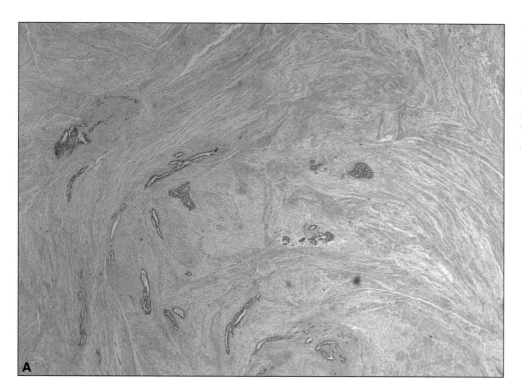

Figure 4.4. Extensive myoid metaplasia in the stroma of a fibroadenoma. (A) The stroma in this fibroadenoma was nearly replaced by a spindle population of cells with a distinct muscle-like appearance.

pericanalicular pattern of growth with a hypercellular stroma and florid epithelial hyperplasia (Figure 4.5). Although the stroma is hypercellular, there is no significant stromal atypia, mitotic rate (generally less than 3/10 hpfs) is low, and the borders are circumscribed. Juvenile fibroadenomas, like usual fibroadenomas, can recur and there

Figure 4.4. *(continued)*
Immunohistochemistry for
desmin (B) and smooth
muscle actin (C) confirming
the myoid nature of the
stroma in the lesion shown
in A.

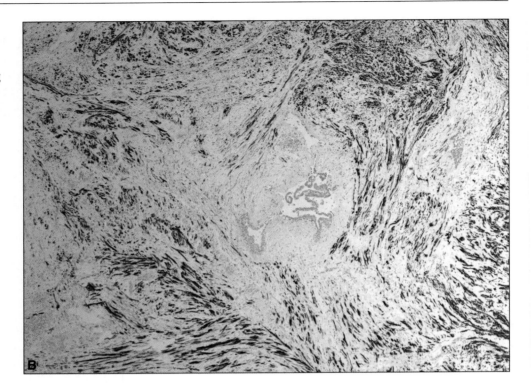

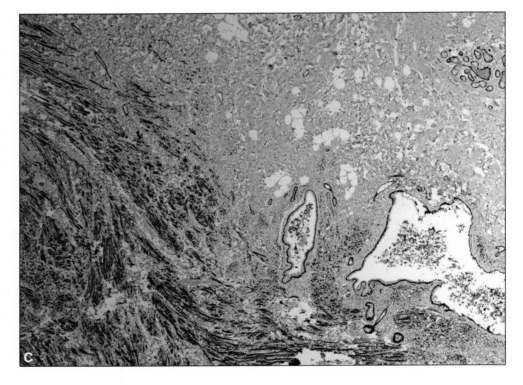

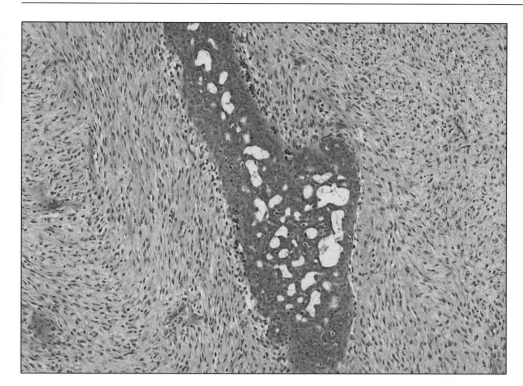

Figure 4.5. Juvenile fibroadenoma. Cellular stroma with rare mitoses and florid ductal epithelial hyperplasia in a fourteen-year old girl.

Table 4.1. Subclassification of Phyllodes Tumors

	Benign	Borderline	Malignant
# of mitoses/10hpfs	0-3	4-9	10 or more
Stromal cellularity and atypia	Mild	Moderate	Marked
Tumor interface	Circumscribed	May be infiltrative	Usually infiltrative
Stromal overgrowth	Absent	May be present	Often present

are reports of multiple, recurring juvenile fibroadenomas occurring particularly in African-American teenage girls.

PHYLLODES TUMOR

Phyllodes tumors are a distinct type of fibroepithelial lesion typically seen in an older age group than fibroadenomas. Grossly, they do not appear significantly different than fibroadenomas and imaging findings are nonspecific although frequently more cystic areas can be seen suggesting phyllodes tumor over fibroadenoma. However, histologic confirmation is required for this distinction.

Microscopically, phyllodes tumors can take on a broad range of appearances. As in fibroadenomas, the tumors are composed of a mixture of stromal and epithelial elements; however, it is the stroma that distinguishes phyllodes tumors from fibroadenomas and also determines the subclassification. Unfortunately, there is neither

Figure 4.6. Benign phyllodes tumor. A circumscribed tumor with leaf-like growth into a cystic space (A,B) with mild stromal cellularity without significant stromal atypia or mitotic activity (C).

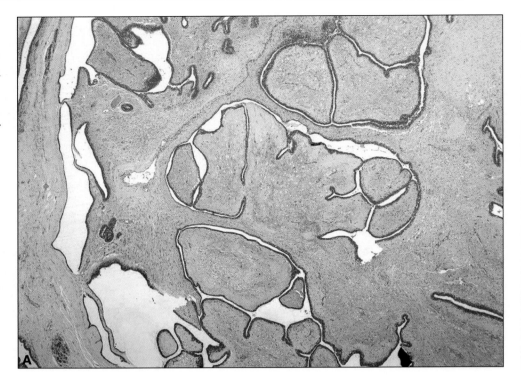

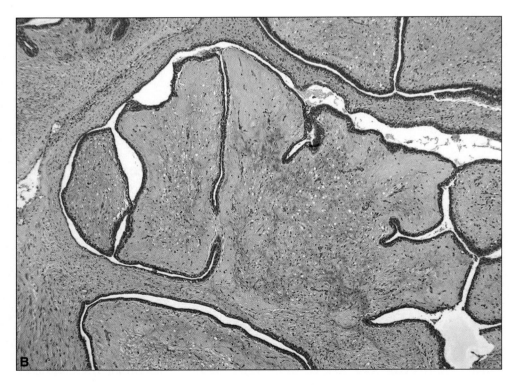

a uniformly agreed subclassification system nor a particular criterion to aid in subclassifying these tumors. A commonly used system separates phyllodes tumors into benign, borderline, and malignant (Table 4.1) based on a set of four histologic criteria (stromal cellularity and atypia, mitotic activity, presence or absence of

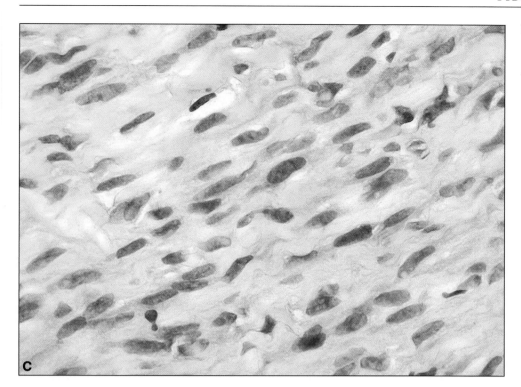

Figure 4.6. *(continued)*

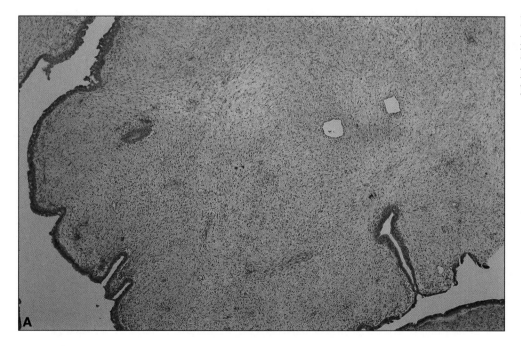

Figure 4.7. Borderline phyllodes tumor. This tumor has a similar leaf-like growth pattern as the benign phyllodes tumor (A);

stromal overgrowth, and character of the tumor border). Benign phyllodes tumors have the characteristic leaf-like growth of phyllodes tumors, with a mild degree of stromal cellularity, low mitotic rate (0–3/hpfs), circumscribed borders, and a lack of stromal overgrowth, which is defined as a full 40× field of pure stroma devoid of

Figure 4.7. *(continued)* however, there is greater stromal cellularity (B), more appreciable stromal atypia, and an increased mitotic rate in the stroma (C).

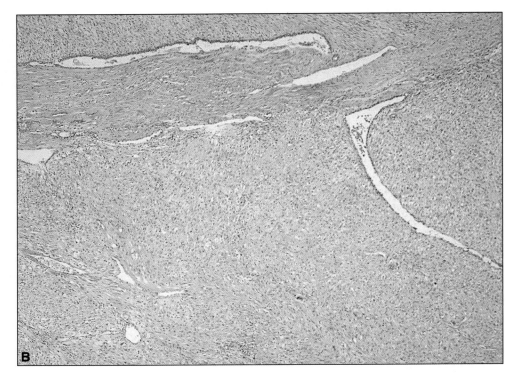

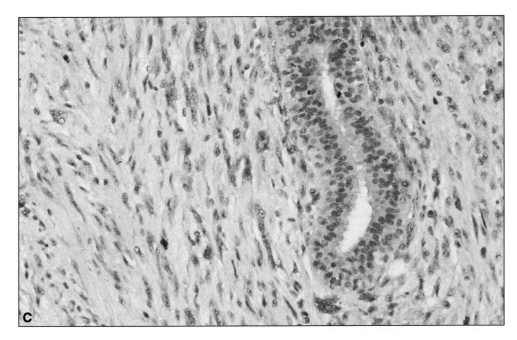

epithelial elements (Figures 4.6A–C). Borderline phyllodes tumors have more cellular stroma with stromal atypia, higher mitotic rates (approximately 4–9/10 hpfs), and sometimes have infiltrative borders, but usually lack stromal overgrowth (Figures 4.7A–C). Malignant phyllodes tumors typically have outright sarcomatous stroma

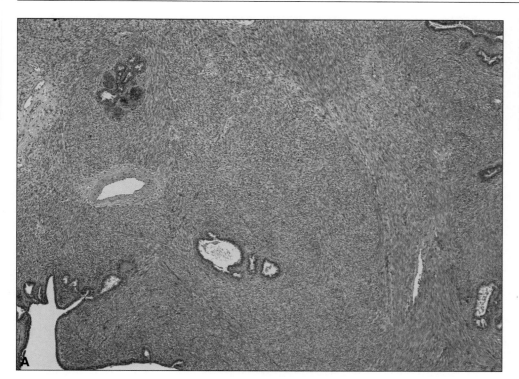

Figure 4.8. Malignant phyllodes tumor. This high-grade tumor maintains leaf-like architecture but there is marked stromal cellularity and atypia and a high mitotic rate (A,B).

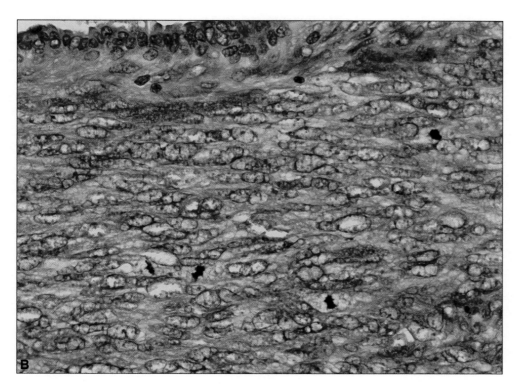

with mitotic activity generally greater than 10/10hpfs, usually have infiltrative bor-ders, and can have stromal overgrowth (Figures 4.8A,B). In several studies, the presence of stromal overgrowth is the feature most associated with aggressive (metastatic) behavior.

Figure 4.9. Fibroadenomas with borderline features. These tumors are circumscribed but have foci in which there is more pronounced intracanalicular growth, cleft-like spaces with periductal condensation, and few mitotic figures (1–2/10hpfs) (A–C).

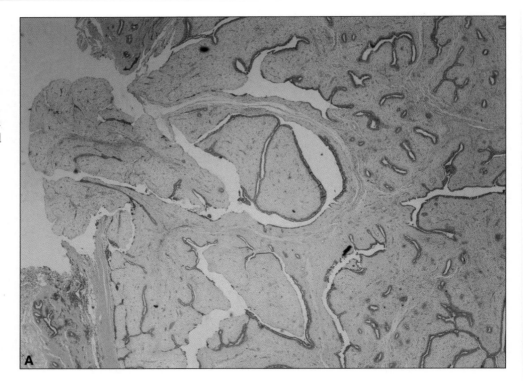

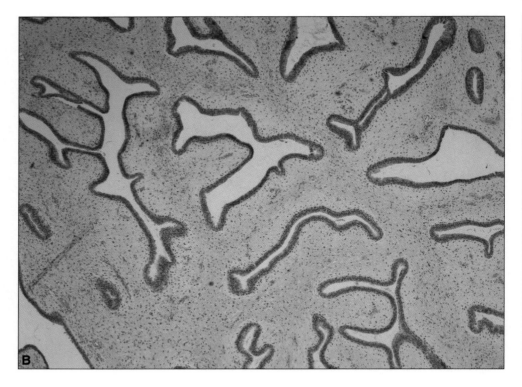

All phyllodes tumors, regardless of subclassification, can recur and generally the rate of recurrence increases from benign to borderline and malignant. Metatases are uncommon and typically associated with the malignant category. Recurrence rates appear to be strongly associated with inadequate surgical margins, as many of these

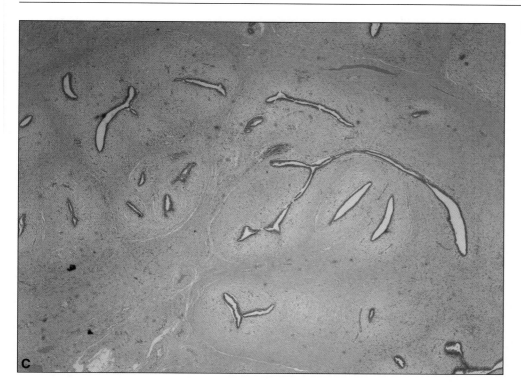

Figure 4.9. (continued)

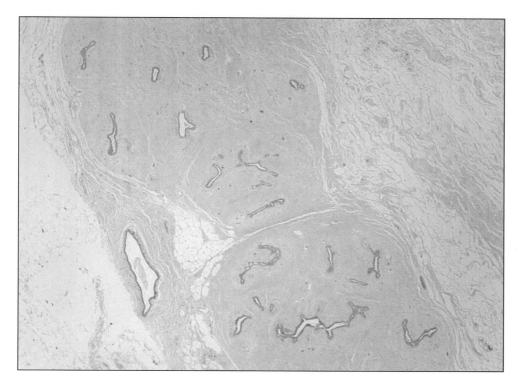

Figure 4.10. Hyalnized fibroadenoma on core needle biopsy. This biopsy was done for a mass lesion and a clear-cut diagnosis of hyalinized fibroadenoma can be made based upon the classic intracanalicular growth pattern and lack of stromal cellularity or atypia.

tumors are "shelled out" surgically as they are preoperatively felt to be fibroade-nomas. Some surgical literature suggests a 1 cm margin of normal tissue surrounding a phyllodes tumor to reduce the risk of recurrence. Numerous studies have looked at immunohistochemical stains as possible prognostic/predictive markers,

Figure 4.11. (A–C) Fibroepithelial lesion on core biopsy with a pericanalicular growth pattern. There is an increase in stromal cellularity without significant atypia but with few mitotic figures. A diagnosis of fibroepithelial lesion, which cannot rule out phyllodes, is made such that a surgical excision for definitive diagnosis can be performed. (D,E) Another fibroepithelial lesion on core biopsy with an intracanalicular growth pattern. This lesion had a milder increase in cellularity than a usual fibroadenoma as well as recognizable stromal mitotic activity. A similar diagnosis of fibroepithelial lesion, cannot rule out phyllodes tumor, is made.

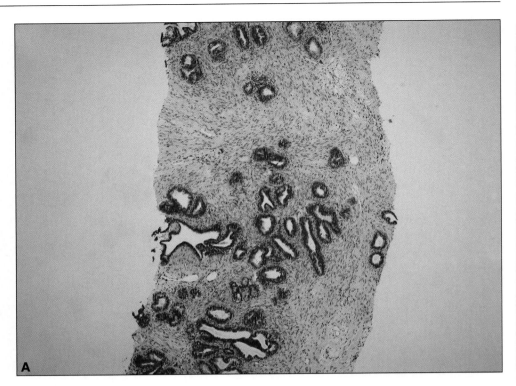

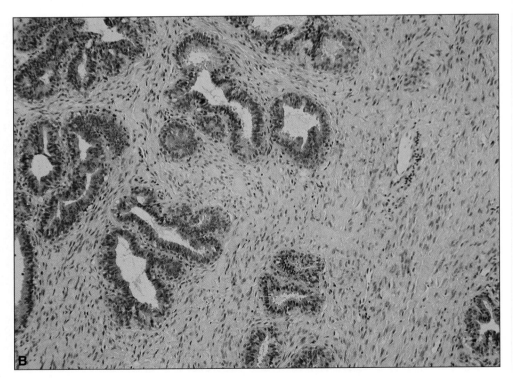

with ki-67 and p53 being the more commonly studied markers. Although many of these markers correlate with the histologic subclassification, very few studies have shown a strong predictive or prognostic role for these markers and thus we do not recommend their use in everyday practice.

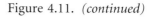

Figure 4.11. *(continued)*

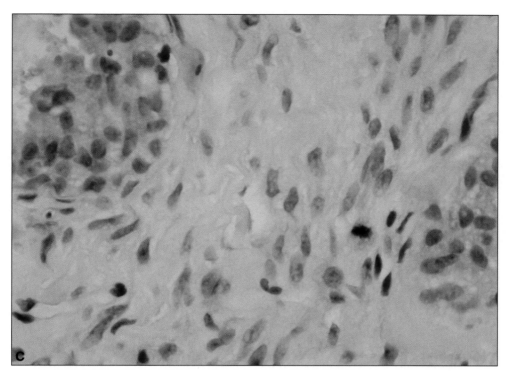

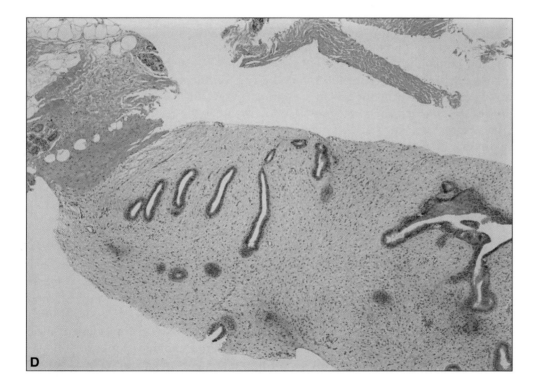

The main differential for phyllodes tumor on the benign end of the spectrum is fibroadenoma. In general, fibroadenomas have a more homogeneous stroma that is not cellular and lacks appreciable mitotic activity; however, some cases show a more pronounced intracanalicular pattern of growth with "cleft-like" spaces and

Figure 4.11. *(continued)*

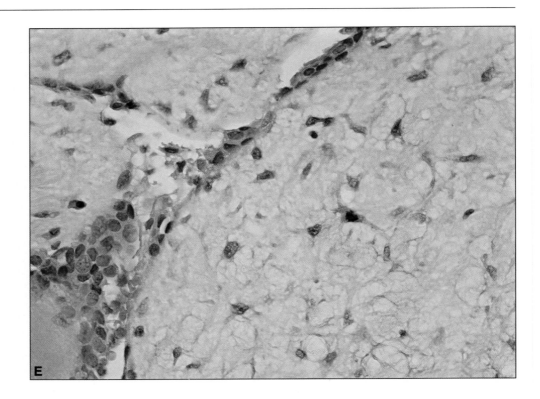

periglandular condensation raising the possibility of a phyllodes tumor (Figures 4.9A–C). Adequate sampling of the lesion to look for areas of more phyllodes-like growth may aid in making this distinction. However, often a clear-cut distinction cannot be made and in those cases we recommend erring on the conservative side and diagnosing cellular fibroadenoma with a comment about the inability to entirely rule out phyllodes tumor and recommend close follow-up as the recurring potential of the lesion is not known. On the malignant end, the differential is with metaplastic carcinoma or sarcoma. Careful sampling to look for any foci of invasive carcinoma, and using NST and/or keratin immunostaining, can aid in this distinction. The finding of "leaf-like" growth does not rule out metaplastic carcinoma. Primary sarcomas of the breast are extremely rare and often occur as part of the stroma of a malignant phyllodes tumor.

With the popularity of core needle biopsy for initial diagnoses of mass lesions, pathologists can be faced with fibroepithelial lesions on core biopsy that cannot be reliably diagnosed as benign fibroadenoma. Although it is straightforward to make a definitive diagnosis when presented with a hyalinized fibroadenoma on core biopsy (Figure 4.10), some lesions may have increased stromal cellularity and may contain stromal mitoses. Since lesions suspected of being phyllodes tumors need to be surgically excised for definitive diagnosis, this is an important clinical distinction. There are only a few studies in the literature that have looked at cellular fibroepithelial lesions on core biopsy. Although there are no uniformly agreed cutoff criteria, in general, a moderate increase in stromal cellularity and the finding of stromal mitotic activity on core biopsy should raise concern for the possibility of phyllodes tumor and a recommendation of surgical excision should be made (Figures 4.11A–E).

REFERENCES

Barth, R. J., Jr. (1999). "Histologic features predict local recurrence after breast conserving therapy of phyllodes tumors." *Breast Cancer Res Treat* 57(3): 291–5.

Ben Hassouna, J., T. Damak, et al. (2006). "Phyllodes tumors of the breast: a case series of 106 patients." *Am J Surg* 192(2): 141–7.

Carter, B. A. and D. L. Page (2004). "Phyllodes tumor of the breast: local recurrence versus metastatic capacity." *Hum Pathol* 35(9): 1051–2.

Chaney, A. W., A. Pollack, et al. (2000). "Primary treatment of cystosarcoma phyllodes of the breast." *Cancer* 89(7): 1502–11.

Chen, W. H., S. P. Cheng, et al. (2005). "Surgical treatment of phyllodes tumors of the breast: retrospective review of 172 cases." *J Surg Oncol* 91(3): 185–94.

Chu, J. S., K. J. Chang, et al. (1995). "Clinicopathologic study of phyllodes tumor of the breast." *J Formos Med Assoc* 94(5): 238–42.

Ciatto, S., R. Bonardi, et al. (1992). "Phyllodes tumor of the breast: a multicenter series of 59 cases. Coordinating Center and Writing Committee of FONCAM (National Task Force for Breast Cancer), Italy." *Eur J Surg Oncol* 18(6): 545–9.

Cohn-Cedermark, G., L. E. Rutqvist, et al. (1991). "Prognostic factors in cystosarcoma phyllodes. A clinicopathologic study of 77 patients." *Cancer* 68(9): 2017–22.

Daniel, W. A., Jr. and M. D. Mathews (1968). "Tumors of the breast in adolescent females." *Pediatrics* 41(4): 743–9.

de Roos, W. K., P. Kaye, et al. (1999). "Factors leading to local recurrence or death after surgical resection of phyllodes tumours of the breast." *Br J Surg* 86(3): 396–9.

Dupont, W. D., D. L. Page, et al. (1994). "Long-term risk of breast cancer in women with fibroadenoma." *N Engl J Med* 331(1): 10–15.

Eroglu, E., C. Irkkan, et al. (2004). "Phyllodes tumor of the breast: case series of 40 patients." *Eur J Gynaecol Oncol* 25(1): 123–5.

Fajdic, J., N. Gotovac, et al. (2007). "Phyllodes tumors of the breast diagnostic and therapeutic dilemmas." *Onkologie* 30(3): 113–18.

Fekete, P., J. Petrek, et al. (1987). "Fibroadenomas with stromal cellularity. A clinicopathologic study of 21 patients." *Arch Pathol Lab Med* 111(5): 427–32.

Geisler, D. P., M. J. Boyle, et al. (2000). "Phyllodes tumors of the breast: a review of 32 cases." *Am Surg* 66(4): 360–6.

Grimes, M. M. (1992). "Cystosarcoma phyllodes of the breast: histologic features, flow cytometric analysis, and clinical correlations." *Mod Pathol* 5(3): 232–9.

Hart, W. R., R. C. Bauer, et al. (1978). "Cystosarcoma phyllodes. A clinicopathologic study of twenty-six hypercellular periductal stromal tumors of the breast." *Am J Clin Pathol* 70(2): 211–16.

Hawkins, R. E., J. B. Schofield, et al. (1992). "The clinical and histologic criteria that predict metastases from cystosarcoma phyllodes." *Cancer* 69(1): 141–7.

Inoshita, S. (1988). "Phyllodes tumor (cystosarcoma phyllodes) of the breast. A clinicopathologic study of 45 cases." *Acta Pathol Jpn* 38(1): 21–33.

Jacobs, T. W., Y. Y. Chen, et al. (2005). "Fibroepithelial lesions with cellular stroma on breast core needle biopsy: are there predictors of outcome on surgical excision?" *Am J Clin Pathol* 124(3): 342–54.

Kario, K., S. Maeda, et al. (1990). "Phyllodes tumor of the breast: a clinicopathologic study of 34 cases." *J Surg Oncol* 45(1): 46–51.

Komenaka, I. K., M. El-Tamer, et al. (2003). "Core needle biopsy as a diagnostic tool to differentiate phyllodes tumor from fibroadenoma." *Arch Surg* 138(9): 987–90.

Kuijper, A., E. C. Mommers, et al. (2001). "Histopathology of fibroadenoma of the breast." *Am J Clin Pathol* 115(5): 736–42.

Lee, A. H., Z. Hodi, et al. (2007). "Histological features useful in the distinction of phyllodes tumour and fibroadenoma on needle core biopsy of the breast." *Histopathology* 51(3): 336–44.

Mangi, A. A., B. L. Smith, et al. (1999). "Surgical management of phyllodes tumors." *Arch Surg* 134(5): 487–92; discussion 492-3.

Moffat, C. J., S. E. Pinder, et al. (1995). "Phyllodes tumours of the breast: a clinicopathological review of thirty-two cases." *Histopathology* 27(3): 205–18.

Murad, T. M., J. R. Hines, et al. (1988). "Histopathological and clinical correlations of cystosarcoma phyllodes." *Arch Pathol Lab Med* 112(7): 752–6.

Norris, H. J. and H. B. Taylor (1967). "Relationship of histologic features to behavior of cystosarcoma phyllodes. Analysis of ninety-four cases." *Cancer* 20(12): 2090–9.

Pietruszka, M. and L. Barnes (1978). "Cystosarcoma phyllodes: a clinicopathologic analysis of 42 cases." *Cancer* 41(5): 1974–83.

Pike, A. M. and H. A. Oberman (1985). "Juvenile (cellular) adenofibromas. A clinicopathologic study." *Am J Surg Pathol* 9(10): 730–6.

Rajan, P. B., M. L. Cranor, et al. (1998). "Cystosarcoma phyllodes in adolescent girls and young women: a study of 45 patients." *Am J Surg Pathol* 22(1): 64–9.

Reinfuss, M., J. Mitus, et al. (1996). "The treatment and prognosis of patients with phyllodes tumor of the breast: an analysis of 170 cases." *Cancer* 77(5): 910–16.

Remadi, S., A. Ismail, et al. (1994). "[Cellular (juvenile) fibroadenoma of the breast. A clinicopathologic and immunohistochemical study of 7 cases]." *Ann Pathol* 14(6): 392–7.

Roa, J. C., O. Tapia, et al. (2006). "Prognostic factors of phyllodes tumor of the breast." *Pathol Int* 56(6): 309–14.

Salvadori, B., F. Cusumano, et al. (1989). "Surgical treatment of phyllodes tumors of the breast." *Cancer* 63(12): 2532–6.

Taira, N., D. Takabatake, et al. (2007). "Phyllodes tumor of the breast: stromal overgrowth and histological classification are useful prognosis-predictive factors for local recurrence in patients with a positive surgical margin." *Jpn J Clin Oncol* 37(10): 730–6.

Tan, E. Y., P. H. Tan, et al. (2006). "Recurrent phyllodes tumours of the breast: pathological features and clinical implications." *ANZ J Surg* 76(6): 476–80.

Tan, P. H. (2005). "2005 Galloway Memorial Lecture: Breast phyllodes tumours – morphology and beyond." *Ann Acad Med Singapore* 34(11): 671–7.

Tan, P. H., T. Jayabaskar, et al. (2005). "Phyllodes tumors of the breast: the role of pathologic parameters." *Am J Clin Pathol* 123(4): 529–40.

Tavassoli, F. (1999). *Biphasic Tumors. Pathology of the Breast.* F. Tavassoli. Stamford, CT, Appleton and Lange: 571–631.

Treves, N. and D. A. Sunderland (1951). "Cystosarcoma phyllodes of the breast: a malignant and a benign tumor; a clinicopathological study of seventy-seven cases." *Cancer* 4(6): 1286–1332.

Ward, R. M. and H. L. Evans (1986). "Cystosarcoma phyllodes. A clinicopathologic study of 26 cases." *Cancer* 58(10): 2282–9.

5 NIPPLE LESIONS

Carol Reynolds, MD

Paget's Disease of the Nipple	55
Nipple Adenoma	57
Syringomatous Adenoma	64

PAGET'S DISEASE OF THE NIPPLE

Paget's disease of the nipple is believed to be a manifestation of comedo-type ductal carcinoma in situ (DCIS), which when involving the subareolar ducts can extend within the confines of the duct and epidermal basement membrane into the epidermis. This is supported by the identification of high-grade DCIS in at least one subareolar nipple duct in most of the cases. Approximately 35–50 percent of patients with Paget's disease of the nipple will have an invasive mammary carcinoma. Paget's disease occurs in approximately 2 percent of patients with breast cancer.

Clinical Features

Clinically, patients present with an erythematous or eczematous rash of the nipple. This clinical picture may be indistinguishable from eczema or other chronic forms of dermatitis.

Macroscopic/Microscopic Features

The nipple skin shows an erythematous or eczematous eruption, which can be crusted or scaly. Histologically, the nipple epidermis shows an infiltrate of single or small groups of large pleomorphic tumor cells (Figure 5.1). These tumor cells have abundant clear-staining cytoplasm, some of which may be vacuolated (Figure 5.2). There is usually an accompanying lymphocytic infiltrate and the overlying epidermis may be hyperplastic and show parakeratosis. The tumor cells show positive staining for periodic acid Schiff (PAS) diastase–resistant mucins; however, immunohistochemistry appears to be a more sensitive method for diagnosis. Paget cells stain positively for the low-molecular-weight cytokeratin (CAM5.2) (Figure 5.3). Amplification of the oncogene HER2 has been associated with high-

Figure 5.1. Paget's disease of the nipple. Malignant glandular epithelial cells forming a band in the deep epidermis. Paget cells also scattered within the epidermis.

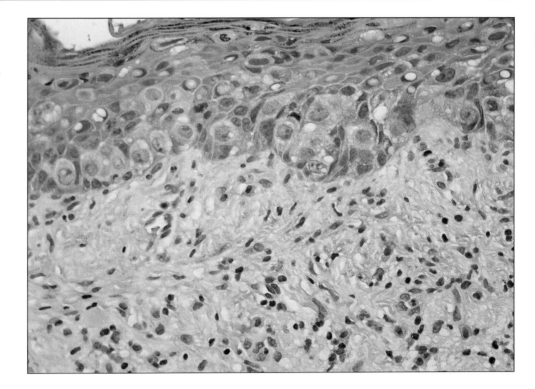

Figure 5.2. Paget cells. The tumor cells are large and pleomorphic with abundant eosinophilic cytoplasm and prominent nucleoli.

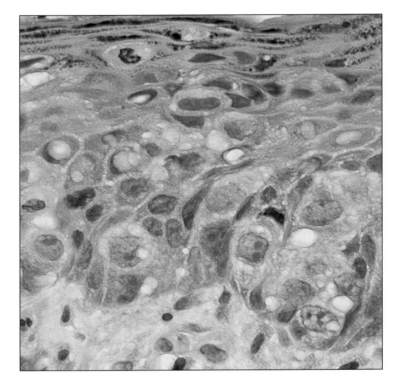

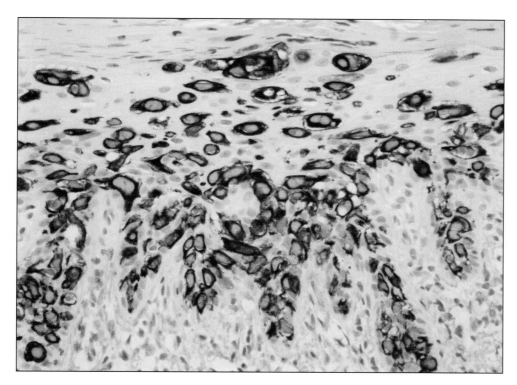

Figure 5.3. Cytokeratin 7. The cytoplasm of the Paget cells are highlighted by cytokeratin 7. The squamous cells are negative for cytokeratin 7 (Contributed by Dr. Lori A. Erickson).

nuclear-grade DCIS and occurs in more than 90 percent of Paget's disease of the nipple, which can also be useful for diagnosis (Figure 5.4) (Table 5.1).

Differential Diagnosis

Clinically, Paget's disease can mimic erosive papillomatosis (nipple adenoma). However, histologically, these two entities do not cause diagnostic difficulty. The large pleomorphic cells in the nipple epidermis may prove difficult to be distinguished from melanocytes, Toker cells, or atypical keratinocytes. Immunohistochemistry together with cytology will be very helpful in discriminating these entities. In a severely inflamed nipple, it may also be difficult to identify the infiltrate of the neoplastic cells. Immunohistochemistry is the preferred method for demonstration of Paget's disease.

Treatment and Prognosis

Treatment is based on the extent of the associated carcinoma.

NIPPLE ADENOMA

The term nipple adenoma is not a specific entity, but has been used to describe any mass lesion of the nipple that is benign. These lesions are known by several different terms (erosive papillomatosis, papillary adenoma, and florid or subareolar

Figure 5.4. HER2. Cytoplasmic membrane staining for HER2 protein outlines the Paget cells in the epidermis (Contributed by Dr. Lori A. Erickson).

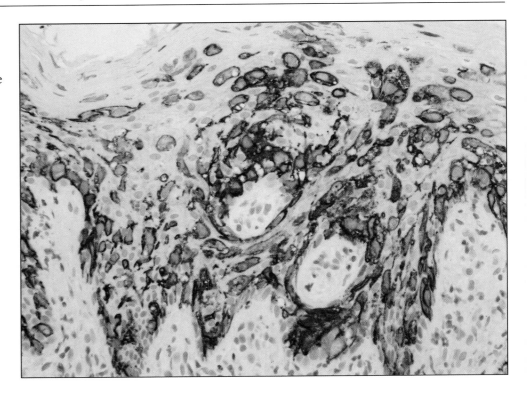

Table 5.1. Paget Cells in Epidermis: Immunophenotypic Features

Immunohistochemical Marker	Mammary Paget's Disease	Squamous Cell Carcinoma	Malignant Melanoma	Toker Cells
CAM5.2	Positive	Negative	Negative	Positive
CK7	Positive	Negative	Negative	Positive
CEA	Positive	Negative	Positive/Negative	Positive
GCDFP-15	Positive	Negative	Negative	Positive/Negative
S-100	Positive/Negative	Negative	Positive	Positive/Negative
HER2	Positive	Negative	Negative	Negative

sclerosing duct papillomatosis) and show a variety of histologic features. Overall, these terms refer to an entity composed of an exuberant proliferation of epithelium, which exhibits both papillary and adenomatous patterns. The first description of nipple adenoma (florid papillomatosis) was published by Jones in 1955.

Clinical Features

Nipple adenomas may occur at any age after puberty and primarily affect women in their fourth and fifth decades. Rarely, these lesions have been described in men. The most common clinical presentation is blood-tinged or serous nipple discharge. Another common symptom is a small firm nodule beneath the nipple. Sometimes, the nipple may be crusted or reddened, mimicking the appearances of Paget's disease. The correct diagnosis is usually established after histological examination.

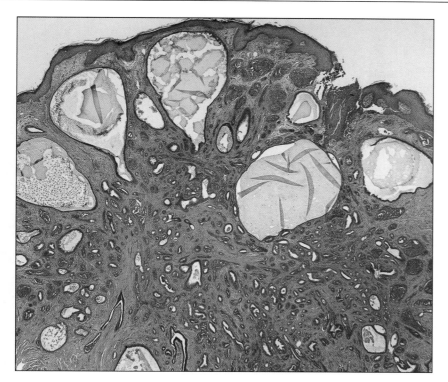

Figure 5.5. Nipple adenoma. Low-power magnification demonstrating a distinct lesion beneath the epidermis composed of adenosis, and epithelial and papillary proliferation.

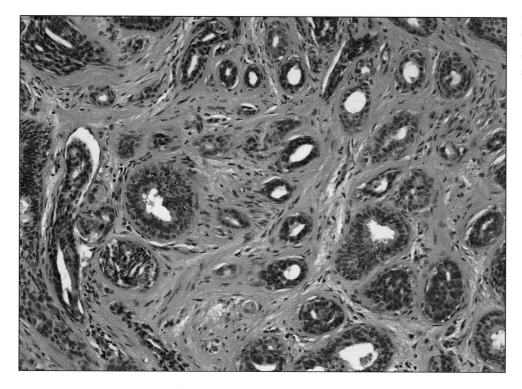

Figure 5.6. Adenosis pattern. The glandular structures are orderly and crowded. There is a distinct two-cell layer.

Macroscopic/Microscopic Features

The size of nipple adenomas range from 1 to 1.5 cm. Grossly, the nipple may be enlarged with overlying skin thickening and sometimes an ill-defined, firm nodule

Figure 5.7. Papillary hyperplasia. Complex epithelial proliferation.

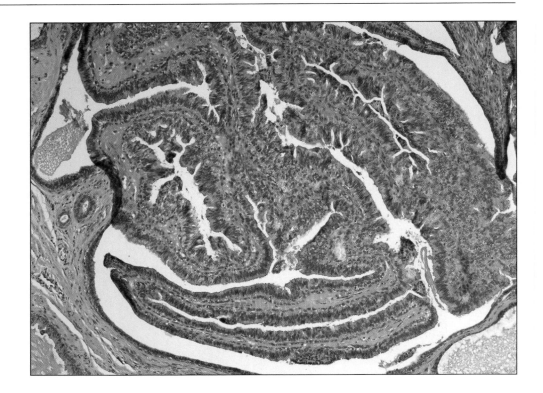

Figure 5.8. Florid ductal hyperplasia. Multiple ducts involved by an exuberant epithelial proliferation.

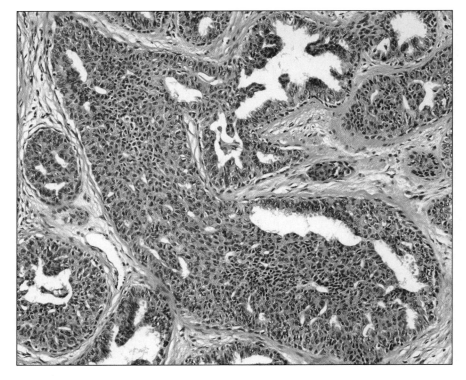

without specific distinguishing features. The histologic features are variable. On low-power examination, a well-circumscribed lesion without encapsulation is seen (Figure 5.5). The main component of this lesion is a diffuse papillary epithelial proliferation (Figures 5.7 and 5.8) intermingled with adenomatous areas composed

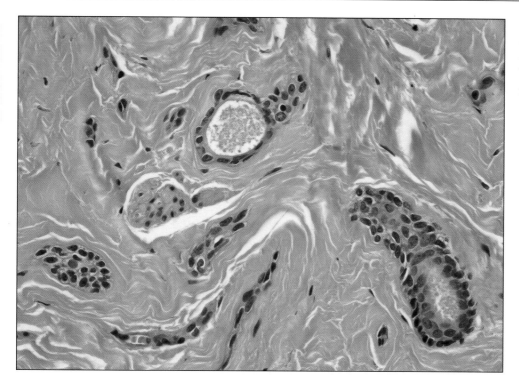

Figure 5.9. Syringomatous adenoma. Numerous nests of epithelial cells intervening between muscle bundles of nipple stroma.

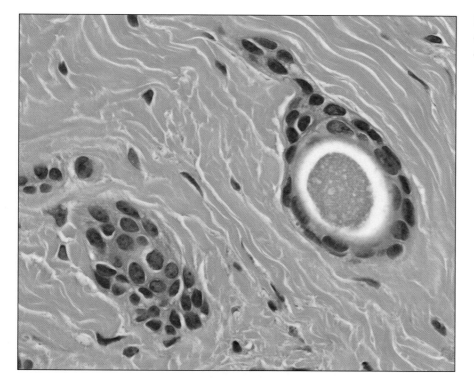

Figure 5.10. Syringomatous epithelium. Cords and nest of cells infiltrating stroma.

of small- and medium-sized glandular structures (Figure 5.6). The epithelial structures have a dual cell population. The presence of two-cell types is a very important feature and immunohistochemical stains for myoepithelial cells can be used to confirm the presence of a myoepithelial layer. The glandular structures may extend

Figure 5.11. Keratinous cysts. Large cysts lined by squamous epithelium.

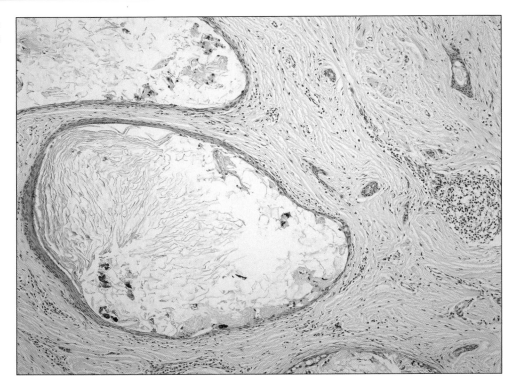

Figure 5.12. Ductules and angulated glands showing characteristic "comma" shape.

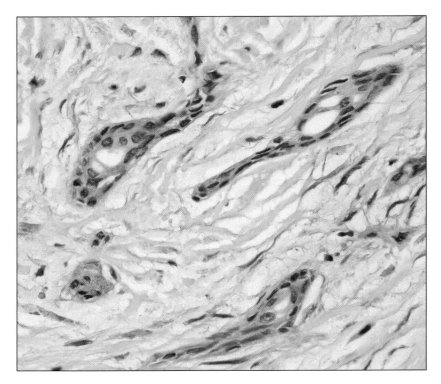

to the surface of the nipple with transition from columnar or cuboidal cells to squamous epithelium. The proliferation seen within the glandular structures varies considerably and may produce a papillary, cribriform, or solid growth pattern. Apocrine metaplasia is common and occasional squamous-lined cysts may be

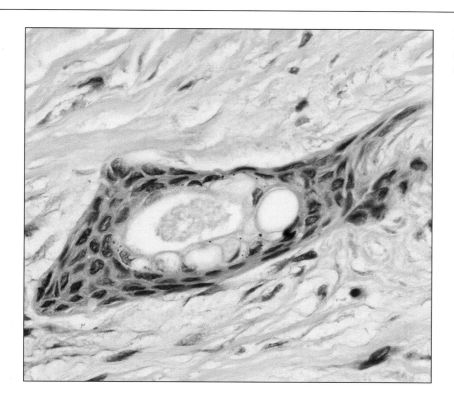

Figure 5.13. Syringomatous glands. Angulated gland with squamoid differentiation.

Table 5.2. Differential Diagnosis of Nipple and Syringomatous Adenomas

Feature	Nipple Adenoma	Syringomatous Adenoma	Tubular Carcinoma	Low-Grade Adenosquamous Carcinoma
Periphery	Smooth circumscription	Infiltrative	Infiltrative	Infiltrative
Lumens	Variable	Angulated, tear drop, comma shaped	Open, angulated	Angulated, tear drop, comma shaped
Myoepithelial layer	Present	Usually present	Absent	Absent
Epithelial proliferation	Present, usually florid	Absent	Absent	Absent
Keratin cyst formation	Often absent	Present	Absent	Present
Apocrine metaplasia	Present	Absent	Absent	Absent
In-situ carcinoma	Absent	Absent	Usually present	Variable
Stroma	Nonreactive	Nonreactive/Reactive	Desmoplastic	Desmoplastic
Potential for metastasis	No	None to date	Yes	Yes

present. Usually, a cellular stroma accompanies the epithelial proliferative process and at the periphery of the lesion, a pseudoinfiltrative pattern of entrapped tubules may be seen. Together with the occasional presence of necrosis, rare mitotic figures within the proliferating epithelium, and the pseudoinfiltrative growth pattern, one should not mistake this as evidence for malignancy.

Differential Diagnosis

Nipple adenomas should be distinguished from the rare tumor syringomatous adenoma and carcinoma. Syringomatous adenoma has an infiltrative growth pattern and lacks circumscription. The small randomly arranged tubules, nests, and cords of epithelial cells intermixed with squamous-lined cysts within a reactive/desmoplastic stroma infiltrate among lactiferous ducts with smooth muscle and perineural invasion (Figures 5.9–5.13). In addition, the tubules in both nipple adenomas and syringomatous adenomas have a dual cell population in contrast to carcinoma (Table 5.2). Atypical ductal hyperplasia as well as carcinoma has been identified in association with nipple adenoma.

Treatment and Prognosis

The lesion is biologically benign and a simple resection is an adequate therapy.

SYRINGOMATOUS ADENOMA

Syringomatous adenoma of the nipple is a rare neoplasm, which has histological features similar to those of eccrine syringoma. The origin of this lesion is unclear. Some authors suggest that syringomatous adenomas may arise from breast parenchyma whereas others believe that they arise from the overlying skin or nipple epidermis and are truly of skin adnexal origin. The major significance of this lesion lies primarily in its recognition as a distinctive benign neoplasm, which should not be mistaken for a malignant tumor.

Clinical Features

Syringomatous adenomas most frequently present as firm, well-defined masses or plaques in the nipple. These lesions have been reported in women and rarely in men.

Macroscopic/Microscopic Features

The size of syringomatous adenomas range from 1 to 3 cm. Grossly, they are poorly defined masses, sometimes with cystic areas visible on the cut surface. Histologically, these lesions show a proliferation of angulated, round, or comma-shaped solid and tubular structures of epithelium infiltrating the fibrous stroma of the nipple. The stroma may be unremarkable or may show edema or even a desmoplastic reactive change. These epithelial structures may extend into the smooth muscle of the nipple. The tubular elements are glandular elements and may show squamous metaplasia. Keratinizing squamous cysts may also be seen. On low-power examination, the tubules are small and inconspicuous, and may be overlooked. These tubular structures have a dual cell population; however, a distinct myoepithelial layer is not typically evident. Mitotic figures are sparse. Several authors have reported these lesions to show perineural invasion, a feature which should not be overinterpreted as indicative of malignancy.

Differential Diagnosis

Syringomatous adenomas may be misdiagnosed as tubular carcinoma, nipple adenoma, or low-grade adenosquamous carcinoma. The tubules of tubular carcinoma lack the dual cell population, which is seen in syringomatous adenomas. In addition, the tubules in tubular carcinomas are smaller and lack squamous differentiation. Nipple adenomas form a well-defined mass, which displaces the nipple stroma rather than the infiltrate. The epithelial proliferation seen in nipple adenomas is more hyperplastic with less stroma seen in between the epithelial islands. Squamous metaplasia can be seen in nipple adenomas as in syringomatous adenomas, but usually the squamous metaplasia is only seen in the superficial portion of the lesion and is not present in the deep portion of the lesion. In syringomatous adenomas, squamous metaplasia can often be prominent throughout the entire lesion. Low-grade adenosquamous carcinomas are similar to infiltrating syringomatous adenomas in that they are composed of solid cords and glandular structures with angulation and infiltrate the breast parenchyma. The stroma in these lesions is frequently desmoplastic. The majority of low-grade adenosquamous carcinomas are reported to be located within the breast parenchyma. However, the differential diagnosis between low-grade adenosquamous carcinoma and infiltrating syringomatous adenoma of the nipple is very difficult, if not impossible, especially when one of the cases in Rosen series is located in the subareolar region.

Treatment and Prognosis

Initial management involves complete excision of the lesion with negative margins. These lesions have a tendency to recur if incompletely excised. There has been no report of distant metastases.

REFERENCES

Paget's Disease of the Nipple

Chaudary MA, Millis RR, Lane EB, Miller NA. Paget's disease of the nipple: a ten year review including clinical, pathological, and immunohistochemical findings. *Breast Cancer Res Treat* 8:139–46, 1986.

Hitchcock A, Topham S, Bell J, Gullick W., Elston CW, Ellis IO. Routine diagnosis of mammary Paget's disease.: a modern approach. *Am J Surg Pathol* 16:58–61, 1992.

Kohler S, Rouse RV, Smoller BR. The differential diagnosis of pagetoid cells in the epidermis. *Mod Pathol* 11:79–92, 1998.

Lundquist K, Kohler S, Rouse RV. Intraepidermal cytokeratin 7 expression is not restricted to Paget cells but is also seen in Toker cells and Merkel cells. *Am J Surg Pathol* 23:212–19, 1999.

Marucci G, Betts CM, Golouh R, Peterse JL, Foschini MP, Eusebi V. Toker cells are probably precursors of Paget cell carcinoma: a morphological and ultrastructural description. *Virchows Arch* 441:117–23, 2002.

Nipple Adenoma

Bhagavan BS, Patchefsky A, Koss LG. Florid subareolar duct papillomatosis (nipple adenoma) and mammary carcinoma: report of three cases. *Hum Pathol* 4:289–95, 1973.

Diaz NM, Palmer JO, Wick MR. Erosive adenomatosis of the nipple: histology, immuno-histology, and differential diagnosis. *Mod Pathol* 5:179–84, 1992.

Doctor VM, Sirsat MV. Florid papillomatosis (adenoma) and other benign tumours of the nipple and areola. *Br J Cancer* 25:1–9, 1971.

Jones DB. Florid papillomatosis of the nipple ducts. *Cancer* 8:315–19, 1955.

Jones MW, Tavassoli FA. Coexistence of nipple duct adenoma and breast carcinoma: a clinicopathologic study of five cases and review of the literature. *Mod Pathol* 8: 633–6, 1995.

Perzin KH, Lattes R. Papillary adenoma of the nipple (florid papillomatosis, adenoma, adenomatosis): a clinicopathologic study. *Cancer* 29:996–1009, 1972.

Rosen PP, Caicco JA. Florid papillomatosis of the nipple: a study of 51 patients, including nine with mammary carcinoma. *Am J Surg Pathol* 10:87–101, 1986.

Rosen PP. Subareolar sclerosing duct hyperplasia of the breast. *Cancer* 59:1927–30, 1987.

Syringomatous Adenoma

Jones MW, Norris HJ, Snyder RC. Infiltrating syringomatous adenoma of the nipple: a clinical and pathological study of 11 cases. *Am J Surg Pathol* 13:197–201, 1989.

Rosen PP. Syringomatous adenoma of the nipple. *Am J Surg Pathol* 7:739–45, 1983.

Suster S, Moran CA, Hurt MA. Syringomatous squamous tumors of the breast. *Cancer* 67:2350–5, 1991.

Ward BE, Cooper PH, Subramony C. Syringomatous tumor of the nipple. *Am J Clin Pathol* 92:692–6, 1989.

Low-Grade Adenosquamous Carcinoma It is Mentioned in the Segment on Syringomatous Adenomas

Rosen PP, Ernsberger D. Low-grade adenosquamous carcinoma: a variant of metaplastic mammary carcinoma. *Am J Surg Pathol* 11:351–8, 1987.

VanHoeven KH, Drudis T, Cranor ML, Erlandson RA, Rosen PP. Low-grade adenosqua-mous carcinoma of the breast: a clinicopathologic study of 32 cases with ultrastruc-tural analysis. *Am J Surg Pathol* 17:248–58, 1993.

6 PAPILLARY LESIONS

Kimberly H. Allison, MD and Thomas J. Lawton, MD

General Clinical and Radiographic Features	67
Intraductal Papilloma	67
Atypical Ductal Hyperplasia and Ductal Carcinoma in situ Involving a Papilloma	70
Intraductal Papillary Carcinoma and Solid Papillary Carcinoma	70
Encysted/Encapsulated Papillary Carcinoma	73
Management of Papillary Lesions	75

GENERAL CLINICAL AND RADIOGRAPHIC FEATURES

Papillary lesions of the breast most often occur in the central subareolar region but also can be more peripherally located. Nipple discharge is one of the most common clinical presentations, especially in cystic, centrally based lesions. Papillomas may present as a palpable mass, and imaging findings include a well-defined, generally smooth-bordered mass, often with a cystic component. Smaller papillomas may be mammographically occult, especially if not associated with calcifications, but may be well visualized with ultrasound. Peripherally based papillomas tend to be smaller and multiple, often discovered incidentally on imaging as multiple nodular masses. Although papillomas can present at any age, women with multiple peripheral papillomas typically present at a younger age (40–50 years) than women with solitary central papillomas (50–60 years). Solid papillary ductal carcinoma in situ and encysted papillary carcinomas tend to occur in older women (60–80 years).

INTRADUCTAL PAPILLOMA

Intraductal papillomas are benign proliferations composed of fibrovascular papillae lined by epithelium with nonneoplastic characteristics. The epithelial layer is supported by an underlying layer of myoepithelial cells that can usually be visualized on

Figure 6.1. (A) Low-power view of an intraductal papilloma, characterized by a proliferation of complex papillae composed of fibrovascular cores lined by a layer of myoepithelial and overlying benign epithelium. These lesions are intraductal, as shown here with a dilated duct encasing the proliferation. (B) A higher power view of the fibrovascular cores of a benign intraductal papilloma. Note the benign epithelium overlying a layer of myoepithelial cells with clear cytoplasm.

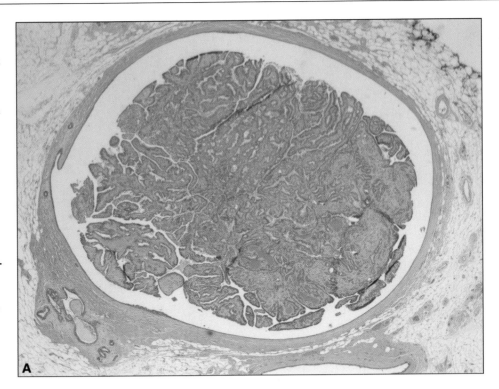

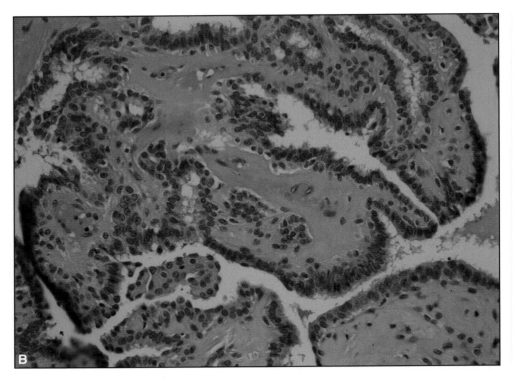

hematoxylin and eosin (H&E) stain as a basal layer of more rounded to spindled cells with paler, frequently clear cytoplasm (Figures 6.1A,B). Immunohistochemical markers such as smooth muscle myosin heavy chain, smooth muscle actin, calponin, and p63, can be useful when the myoepithelial cells are not well visualized in

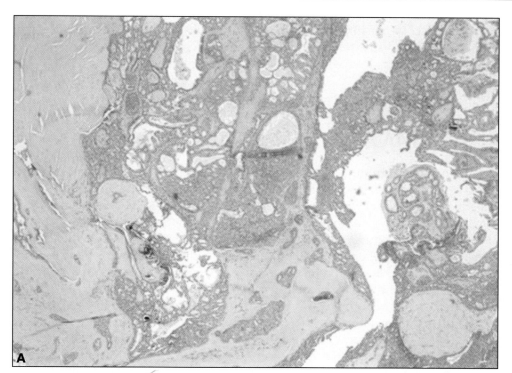

Figure 6.2. (A) Florid hyperplasia and apocrine metaplasia within a sclerosing intraductal papilloma. The extensive sclerosis, common in many papillomas, causes many of the nests of cells to appear infiltrative but this is mere "entrapment." (B) An immunostain for smooth muscle myosin heavy chain, helping to confirm the benign nature of the irregular nests "entrapped" within the sclerosis of the papilloma.

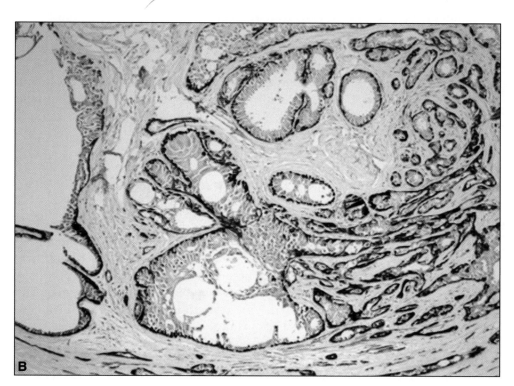

complex cases. Not only are myoepithelial cells present lining the convolutions of the papillae but they are also present lining the surrounding duct. Metaplastic changes are frequent in papillomas, most commonly apocrine and squamous metaplasia. Often, intraductal papillomas are associated with extensive sclerosis giving the appearance of an infiltrative process. Being aware of this finding and using immunohistochemistry for myoepithelial markers in difficult cases can help in confirming the noninvasive nature of a sclerotic papilloma (Figures 6.2A,B).

ATYPICAL DUCTAL HYPERPLASIA AND DUCTAL CARCINOMA IN SITU INVOLVING A PAPILLOMA

The epithelium of an intraductal papilloma often forms just a single layer, but all types of epithelial proliferations can occur within papillomas, including florid hyperplasia of the usual type, atypical ductal hyperplasia (ADH), and ductal carcinoma in situ (DCIS). Although the epithelial proliferations have similar cytologic and architectural features to their counterparts outside of a papilloma, the distinction between these epithelial proliferations can be quite problematic when they arise within papillomas. Some authors have advocated the use of cytokeratin stains, in particular CK5/6 and CK14, to aid in problematic cases distinguishing ADH/DCIS from benign papillomas but this is not particularly useful in separating ADH from DCIS. In addition, although the myoepithelial cells that are typically present throughout a benign intraductal papilloma may be reduced or absent in areas of ADH and DCIS, this does not necessarily help in distinguishing these two entities. Unfortunately, the literature presents conflicting criteria for making the distinction. Some authors have used a more quantitative approach when presented with a case in which a proliferation resembling DCIS is present within a preexisting papilloma. One study advocates a size threshold of >3 mm of involvement by non-high-grade DCIS as diagnostic criteria for a papilloma with DCIS. A similar focus of DCIS occupying ≤3 mm of the papilloma qualifies for a diagnosis of papilloma with ADH. Others advocate a percentage involvement of the papilloma, with a threshold of at least 30 percent involvement by a proliferation qualifying as DCIS before a diagnosis of papilloma with DCIS is rendered (Figures 6.3A,B).

INTRADUCTAL PAPILLARY CARCINOMA AND SOLID PAPILLARY CARCINOMA

In contrast to a papilloma involved by DCIS, intraductal papillary carcinoma is a distinct entity in which the in situ carcinoma grows in a papillary pattern but there is no preexisting/underlying papilloma. These tumors typically have an aborizing papillary growth pattern, but the papillary cores tend to be much thinner and delicate than seen in usual papillomas. One common histology is that of a neoplastic population of columnar-type epithelium, usually one to a few cells thick, lining the thin fibrovascular stalks (Figures 6.4A,B). However, other architectural growth patterns of DCIS can be seen. In intraductal papillary carcinomas, there is no evidence of a myoepithelial cell layer lining the fibrovascular cores (Figures 6.4C,D). However, since this is considered an intraductal lesion, myoepithelium can be identified lining the periphery of the involved duct space.

Solid papillary carcinoma is a unique type of intraductal papillary carcinoma in which the neoplastic cells grow in a solid pattern and the thin fibrovascular cores are often inconspicuous. These tumors may present as multiple large nodules of

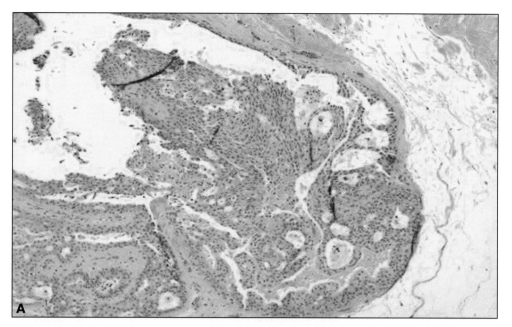

Figure 6.3. (A) Low-power view of a papilloma with atypical ductal hyperplasia. The area of concern occupies less than 30 percent of the overall papilloma and, although cytologically and architecturally worrisome for ductal carcinoma in situ, by convention this is diagnosed as atypical ductal hyperplasia involving a papilloma.
(B) A higher power view of the lesion in Figure 6.3A showing the focal solid proliferation with distinct cell borders concerning for ductal carcinoma in situ. However, the spaces formed are somewhat irregular and there is a layer of residual myoepithelium with clear cytoplasm lining the fibrovascular core.

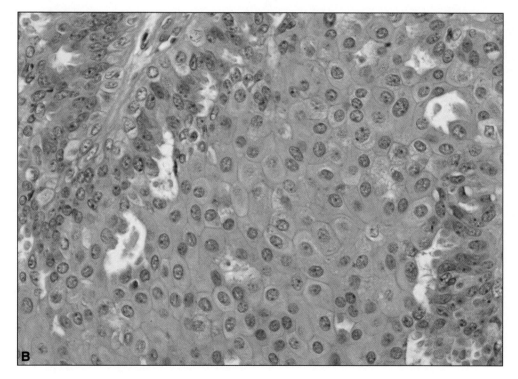

solid papillary growth (Figures 6.5A,B). Often the constituent cells will have a neuroendocrine appearance that can be confirmed by immunohistochemistry (Figure 6.5C); other variants include a spindle-cell type and a clear-cell type. Frequently, intracytoplasmic mucin can be demonstrated in the cells. This finding may be related to the frequent association of this type of papillary intraductal carcinoma with mucinous carcinoma. As is the case with intraductal papillary carcinomas,

Figure 6.4.
(A) A medium-power view of a papillary carcinoma (intraductal). Note the fine fibrovascular cores lined by a layer of columnar-type epithelium with absence of an underlying myoepithelial layer on H&E.
(B) A high-power view of the same lesion showing an absence of myoepithelium lining the fibrovascular cores.
(C) A smooth muscle myosin heavy chain stain showing an absent myoepithelial cell layer lining the fibrovascular cores.
(D) A p63 stain showing complete absence of a myopithelial-cell layer lining the fibrovascular cores.

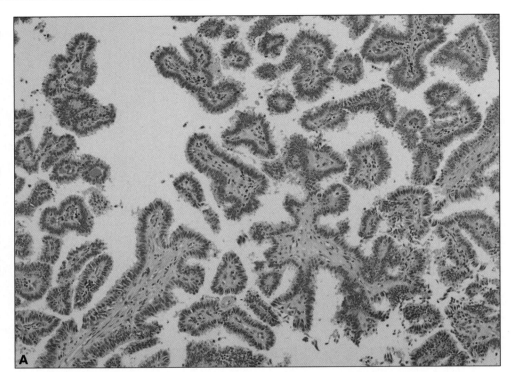

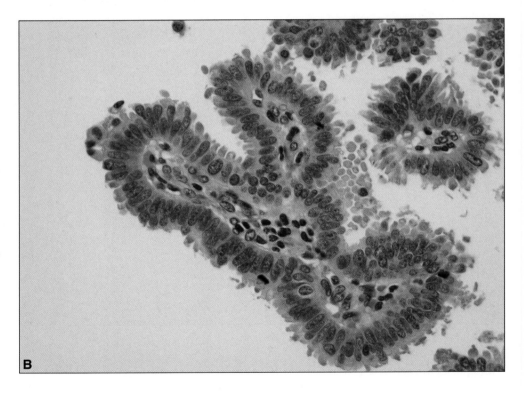

myoepithelial cells are not identified within the tumor. However, in this type of intraductal papillary carcinoma, the data on the presence of myoepithelium around the periphery of some of these tumors is conflicting with some studies indicating a lack of peripheral staining.

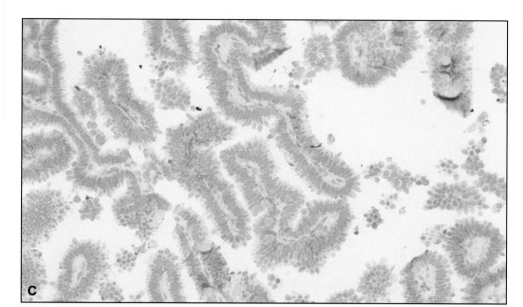

Figure 6.4. *(continued)*

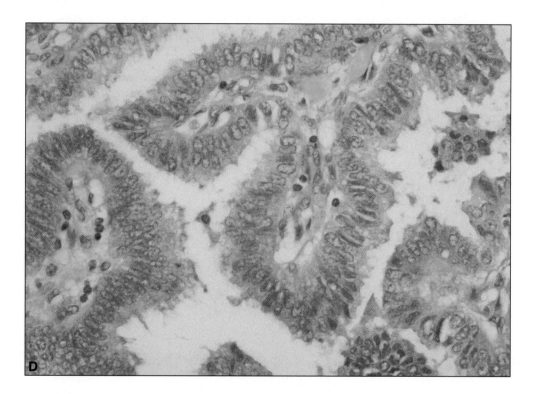

ENCYSTED/ENCAPSULATED PAPILLARY CARCINOMA

This is a unique variant of papillary carcinoma that was originally labeled intracystic papillary carcinoma. The original descriptions were of large papillary carcinomas within cystic ducts, thus the original designation as intracystic. These tumors are frequently large and multinodular in appearance and, although they appear

Figure 6.5. (A) The low-power appearance of solid papillary ductal carcinoma in situ. Note the multinodular growth pattern. Many of these lesions fail to show positive staining for myoepithelial markers at the periphery of the nodules of tumor. (B) Higher power view of solid papillary ductal carcinoma in situ showing a solid growth pattern with fine fibrovascular cores scattered throughout the lesion. (C) High-power view of solid papillary ductal carcinoma in situ showing the uniform cytology with a "neuroendocrine" appearance and polarization of the cells around the fine fibrovascular cores.

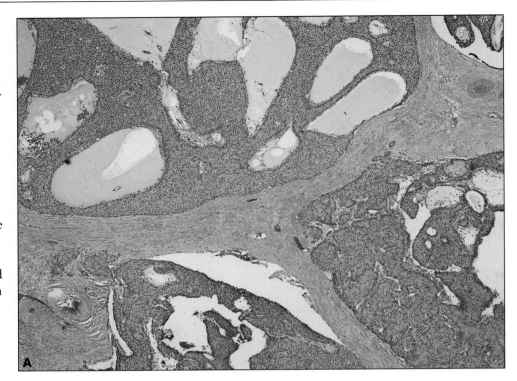

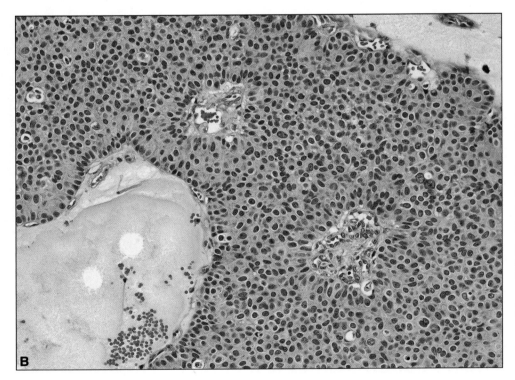

relatively circumscribed, often a discrete peripheral cystically dilated duct is not readily identified (Figure 6.6A). The neoplastic epithelium within the tumor can resemble any of the aforementioned types of DCIS (Figures 6.6B,C). However, based on recent studies showing a lack of myoepithelium at the periphery of these

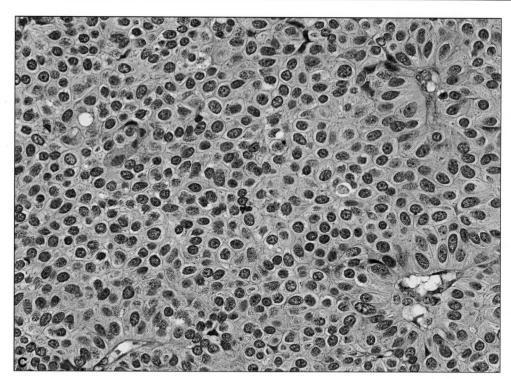

Figure 6.5. *(continued)*

lesions, it is now questionable in the literature as to whether these are truly large intraductal carcinomas or expansile "encysted" invasive carcinomas. In addition, there are rare reports of lymph node metastases associated with this type of papillary carcinoma, lending further evidence that these may in fact be invasive processes (Figure 6.6D).

MANAGEMENT OF PAPILLARY LESIONS

There remains a controversy as to how to manage papillary lesions found at core needle biopsy. Although it is widely accepted that the finding of ADH or DCIS in a papilloma found at core biopsy requires surgical excision, there is still no uniform agreement in the literature as to whether benign intraductal papillomas diagnosed on core biopsy need to be surgically excised. Issues such as size of the sample, size of the lesion by imaging, and correlation with the clinician and breast imagers can aid in making recommendations for the need to surgically excise a benign papilloma diagnosed on core biopsy.

One of the challenges associated with core biopsy, particularly with reference to papillary lesions, is the phenomenon of "epithelial displacement." Due to the unique nature of papillary lesions, often small clusters of cells that appear to be infiltrative can be identified in the biopsy tract following core needle biopsy (Figures 6.7A,B). It is critical to place these cells in perspective and not to overdiagnose invasive carcinoma. The benign appearance of the cell clusters (which often have a squamoid appearance) as well as their presence within the loose fibrosis, fat necrosis, and hemorrhage associated with a prior biopsy site can aid in this distinction.

Figure 6.6. (A) Encysted papillary carcinoma features a papillary neoplastic process with a well-circumscribed, pseudoencapsulated border. (B) Another low-power image of an encysted papillary carcinoma. Although there appears to be a fibrous rim around the lesion, stains for myoepithelium are absent at the periphery. (C) A higher power view of the encysted papillary carcinoma in B. (D). Lymph node with metastatic papillary carcinoma from patient with the encysted papillary carcinoma in Figure 6.6B.

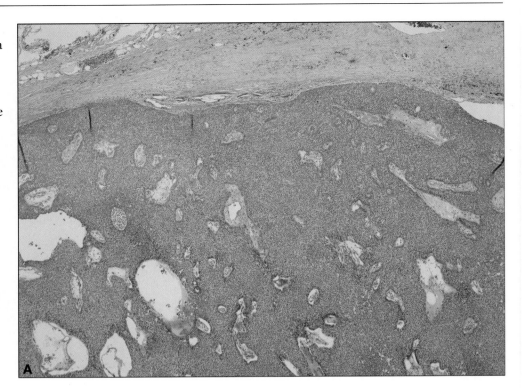

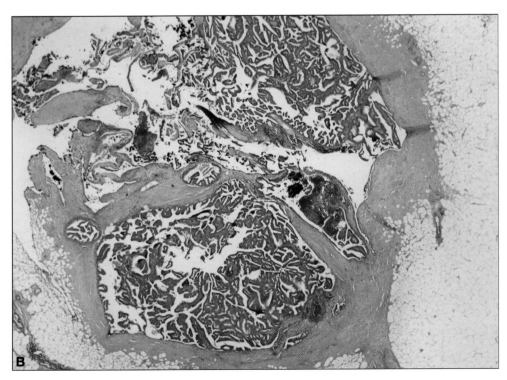

Surgical biopsies containing a papilloma with ADH/DCIS or an intraductal papillary carcinoma should be thoroughly evaluated to determine if there are foci of DCIS or possibly invasive carcinoma in the surrounding tissue. In addition, attention should be paid to margins if DCIS and/or invasive carcinoma is identified.

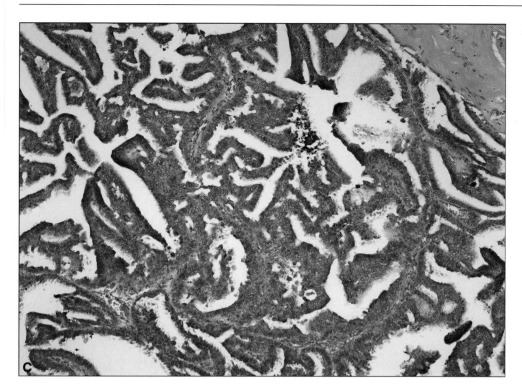

Figure 6.6. *(continued)*

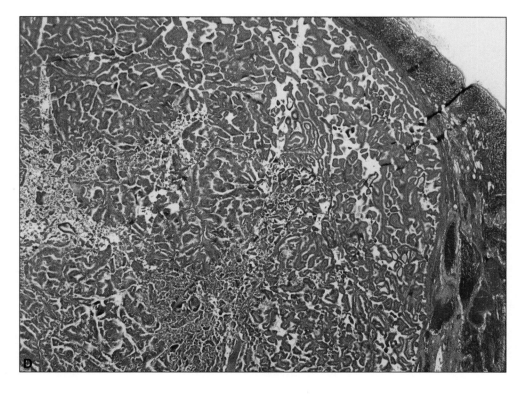

Currently, there is controversy on the recommended management of "encysted" papillary carcinomas. In general, with local therapy alone, these lesions have a favorable prognosis; however, given their staining properties similar to invasive carcinomas and reports of lymph node metastases this recommendation

Figure 6.7. (A) Clusters of epithelial cells haphazardly present within a fibrovascular stroma with associated fat necrosis compatible with epithelial displacement in a biopsy tract. (B) High-power view of the benign-appearing, often squamoid-type clusters of cells within a biopsy tract characteristic of epithelial displacement. These cell clusters should not be confused with invasive carcinoma.

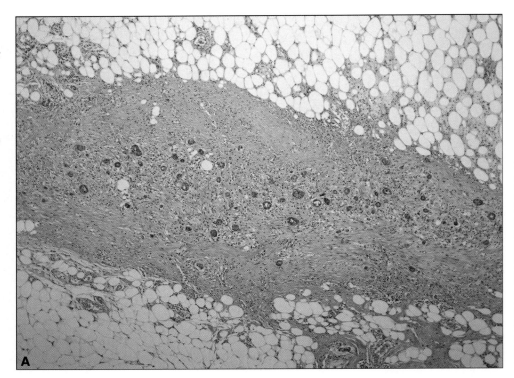

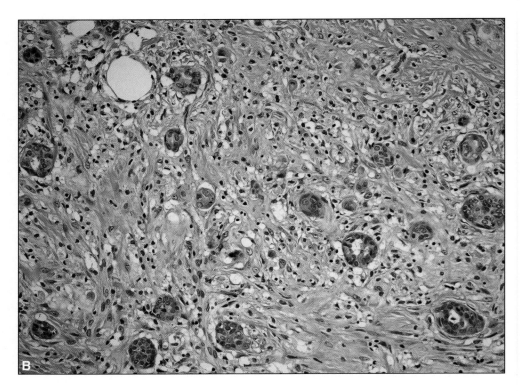

may change. As with intraductal papillary carcinoma, the surrounding tissue should be extensively evaluated to determine if additional foci of DCIS or possibly invasive carcinoma are present and their respective relation to margins noted.

REFERENCES

Agoff, S. N. and T. J. Lawton (2004). "Papillary lesions of the breast with and without atypical ductal hyperplasia: can we accurately predict benign behavior from core needle biopsy?" *Am J Clin Pathol* 122(3): 440–3.

Arora, N., C. Hill, et al. (2007). "Clinicopathologic features of papillary lesions on core needle biopsy of the breast predictive of malignancy." *Am J Surg* 194(4): 444–9.

Carter, D., S. L. Orr, et al. (1983). "Intracystic papillary carcinoma of the breast. After mastectomy, radiotherapy or excisional biopsy alone." *Cancer* 52(1): 14–9.

Collins, L. C., V. P. Carlo, et al. (2006). "Intracystic papillary carcinomas of the breast: a reevaluation using a panel of myoepithelial cell markers." *Am J Surg Pathol* 30(8): 1002–7.

Collins, L. C. and S. J. Schnitt (2008). "Papillary lesions of the breast: selected diagnostic and management issues." *Histopathology* 52(1): 20–9.

Hill, C. B. and I. T. Yeh (2005). "Myoepithelial cell staining patterns of papillary breast lesions: from intraductal papillomas to invasive papillary carcinomas." *Am J Clin Pathol* 123(1): 36–44.

Leal, C., I. Costa, et al. (1998). "Intracystic (encysted) papillary carcinoma of the breast: a clinical, pathological, and immunohistochemical study." *Hum Pathol* 29(10): 1097–104.

Lefkowitz, M., W. Lefkowitz, et al. (1994). "Intraductal (intracystic) papillary carcinoma of the breast and its variants: a clinicopathological study of 77 cases." *Hum Pathol* 25(8): 802–9.

Lewis, J. T., L. C. Hartmann, et al. (2006). "An analysis of breast cancer risk in women with single, multiple, and atypical papilloma." *Am J Surg Pathol* 30(6): 665–72.

Liberman, L., N. Bracero, et al. (1999). "Percutaneous large-core biopsy of papillary breast lesions." *AJR Am J Roentgenol* 172(2): 331–7.

Liberman, L., C. Tornos, et al. (2006). "Is surgical excision warranted after benign, concordant diagnosis of papilloma at percutaneous breast biopsy?" *AJR Am J Roentgenol* 186(5): 1328–34.

MacGrogan, G. and F. A. Tavassoli (2003). "Central atypical papillomas of the breast: a clinicopathological study of 119 cases." *Virchows Arch* 443(5): 609–17.

Maluf, H. M. and F. C. Koerner (1995). "Solid papillary carcinoma of the breast. A form of intraductal carcinoma with endocrine differentiation frequently associated with mucinous carcinoma." *Am J Surg Pathol* 19(11): 1237–44.

Mercado, C. L., D. Hamele-Bena, et al. (2006). "Papillary lesions of the breast at percutaneous core-needle biopsy." *Radiology* 238(3): 801–8.

Moritani, S., S. Ichihara, et al. (2007). "Myoepithelial cells in solid variant of intraductal papillary carcinoma of the breast: a potential diagnostic pitfall and a proposal of an immunohistochemical panel in the differential diagnosis with intraductal papilloma with usual ductal hyperplasia." *Virchows Arch* 450(5): 539–47.

Mulligan, A. M. and F. P. O'Malley (2007). "Papillary lesions of the breast: a review." *Adv Anat Pathol* 14(2): 108–19.

Nagi, C., I. Bleiweiss, et al. (2005). "Epithelial displacement in breast lesions: a papillary phenomenon." *Arch Pathol Lab Med* 129(11): 1465–9.

Nassar, H., H. Qureshi, et al. (2006). "Clinicopathologic analysis of solid papillary carcinoma of the breast and associated invasive carcinomas." *Am J Surg Pathol* 30(4): 501–7.

Page, D. L., K. E. Salhany, et al. (1996). "Subsequent breast carcinoma risk after biopsy with atypia in a breast papilloma." *Cancer* 78(2): 258–66.

Rabban, J. T., F. C. Koerner, et al. (2006). "Solid papillary ductal carcinoma in situ versus usual ductal hyperplasia in the breast: a potentially difficult distinction resolved by cytokeratin 5/6." *Hum Pathol* 37(7): 787–93.

Renshaw, A. A., R. P. Derhagopian, et al. (2004). "Papillomas and atypical papillomas in breast core needle biopsy specimens: risk of carcinoma in subsequent excision." *Am J Clin Pathol* 122(2): 217–21.

Rizzo, M., M. J. Lund, et al. (2008). "Surgical follow-up and clinical presentation of 142 breast papillary lesions diagnosed by ultrasound-guided core-needle biopsy." *Ann Surg Oncol* 15(4): 1040–7.

Rosen, E. L., R. C. Bentley, et al. (2002). "Imaging-guided core needle biopsy of papillary lesions of the breast." *AJR Am J Roentgenol* 179(5): 1185–92.

Sakr, R., R. Rouzier, et al. (2008). "Risk of breast cancer associated with papilloma." *Eur J Surg Oncol.*

Shah, V. I., C. I. Flowers, et al. (2006). "Immunohistochemistry increases the accuracy of diagnosis of benign papillary lesions in breast core needle biopsy specimens." *Histopathology* 48(6): 683–91.

Sydnor, M. K., J. D. Wilson, et al. (2007). "Underestimation of the presence of breast carcinoma in papillary lesions initially diagnosed at core-needle biopsy." *Radiology* 242(1): 58–62.

Tan, P. H., M. Y. Aw, et al. (2005). "Cytokeratins in papillary lesions of the breast: is there a role in distinguishing intraductal papilloma from papillary ductal carcinoma in situ?" *Am J Surg Pathol* 29(5): 625–32.

7 BENIGN STROMAL LESIONS

Thomas J. Lawton, MD

Pseudoangiomatous Stromal Hyperplasia	81
Hemangiomas	81
Hamartoma and Myoid Hamartoma	85
Myofibroblastoma	87
Fibromatosis	89
Granular Cell Tumor	92

PSEUDOANGIOMATOUS STROMAL HYPERPLASIA

Pseudoangiomatous stromal hyperplasia (PASH) can be an incidental finding in breast biopsies or can present as palpable masses. The vast majority of patients are female and premenopausal; however, there are reports of PASH occurring in men, generally in association with gynecomastia. Imaging findings are nonspecific, but usually a mass is seen with circumscribed or partially circumscribed borders; nearly all lack calcifications on mammography.

Microscopically, PASH is composed of anastamosing slit-like spaces in a densely collagenized stroma (Figure 7.1A). The spaces are lined by flat, slender cells that lack cytologic atypia and mitotic activity (Figure 7.1B). The spaces appear vascular and the cells resemble endothelial cells, but immunohistochemistry has shown the constituent cells to be of myofibroblastic origin (positive for vimentin/ CD34/actin and negative for vascular markers). There is no nuclear tufting and the process tends to be lobulocentric but does not "destroy" lobules, which aids in the distinction of PASH from low-grade angiosarcoma.

Surgical excision with clear margins is the recommended treatment. Recurrences have been reported in the literature. Currently, there is no recommendation for treating these lesions with hormonal or radiation therapy.

HEMANGIOMAS

Hemangiomas are benign vascular lesions that can occur as incidental findings or as palpable masses. They can occur at any age and have been reported in men and

Figure 7.1.
(A) Pseudoangiomatous
stromal hyperplasia (PASH).
At low power the
anastamosing slit-like spaces
are seen within a densely
sclerotic stroma.
(B) Higher power view of
PASH surrounding a lobule;
note the bland
myofibroblastic cells lining
the slit-like spaces.

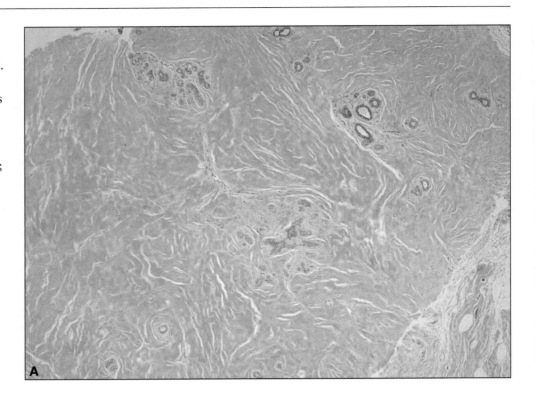

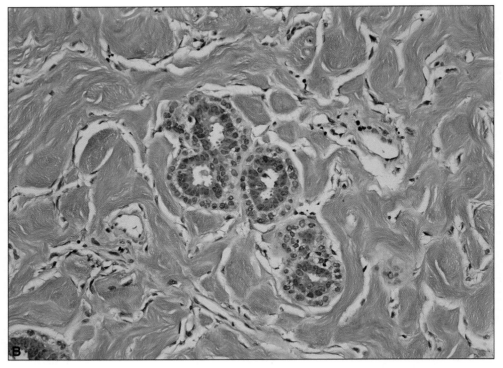

women. On breast imaging, hemangiomas generally appear as lobulated, well-circumscribed masses, which may or may not contain calcifications.

A variety of subtypes of hemangioma occur in the breast and their histology is similar to that in other organ systems. Capillary hemangiomas are generally

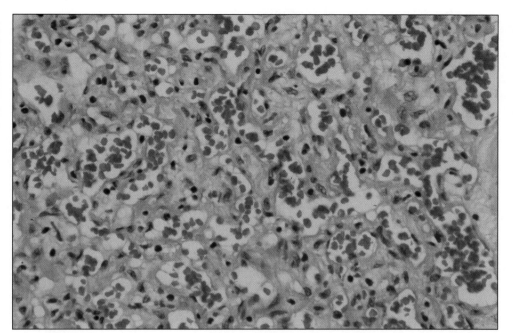

Figure 7.2. Capillary hemangioma composed of a collection of small vascular channels lined by epithelial cells with hyperchromatic nuclei.

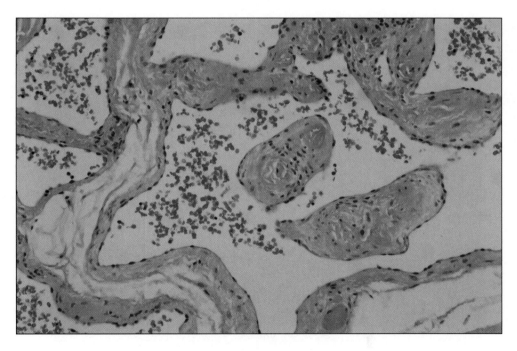

Figure 7.3. Cavernous hemangioma composed of dilated vascular channels lined by flattened endothelial cells. The vascular spaces are filled with red blood cells.

circumscribed lesions composed of a collection of small vessels lined by endothelial cells with hyperchromatic nuclei (Figure 7.2). Cavernous hemangiomas are composed of dilated vascular channels filled with blood and lined by flat endothelial cells (Figure 7.3).

Hemangiomas should be treated by complete local excision. Further treatment is not indicated. There are no reports of recurrences in the literature.

Figure 7.4. (A) Hamartoma, composed of an admixture of fibrous and adipose tissue. Note the circumscribed periphery of the lesion. (B) Higher power view of hamartoma showing the paucicellular fibrous stroma and admixed adipose tissue.

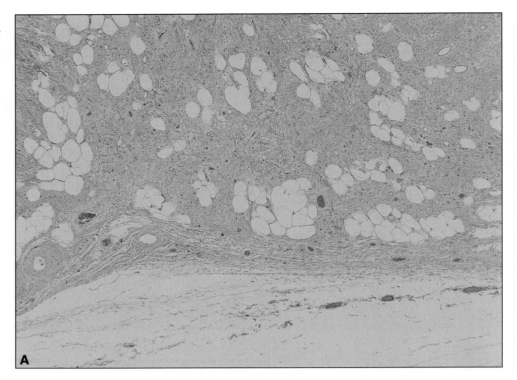

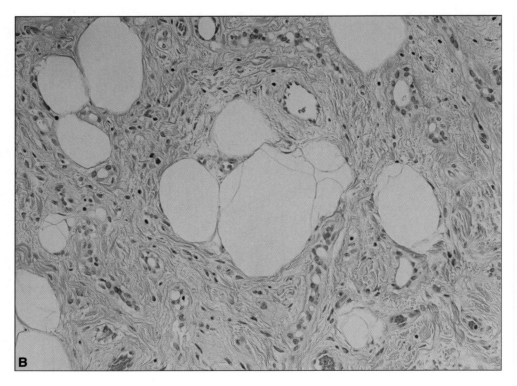

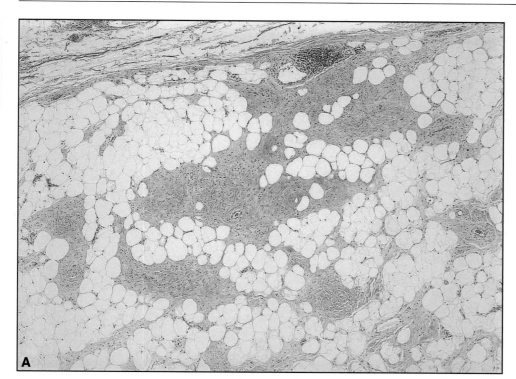

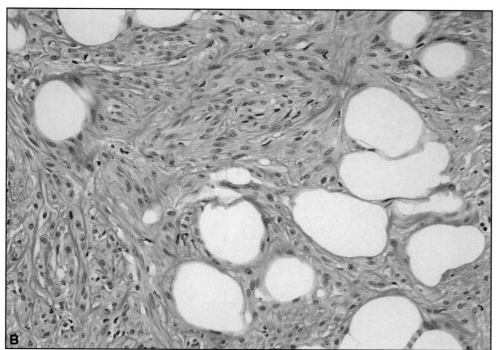

Figure 7.5. (A) Myoid hamartoma. Low-power showing the circumscribed nature of the lesion and admixed fibrous and adipose tissue, the former containing increased cellularity with a "myoid" appearance. (B) High-power view of myoid hamartoma. Note the increased cellularity of the stroma with the characteristic "myoid" appearance.

HAMARTOMA AND MYOID HAMARTOMA

Hamartomas are uncommon lesions, generally presenting as a painless mass in premenopausal women. Imaging generally reveals a circumscribed mass, which can frequently be mistaken for a fibroadenoma.

Figure 7.6.
(A) Myofibroblastoma. The periphery of the lesion is circumscribed. (B,C) The tumor is composed of nests of cells admixed with bands of hyalinized collagen. The constituent cells are round to oval without significant pleomorphism or mitotic activity.

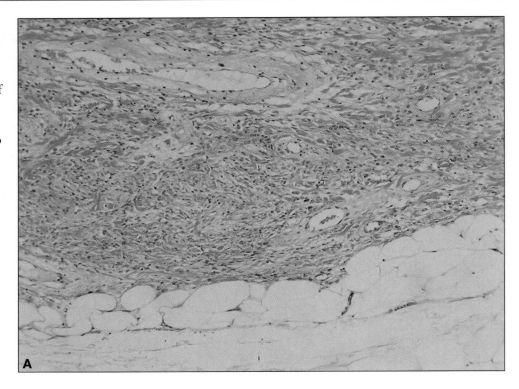

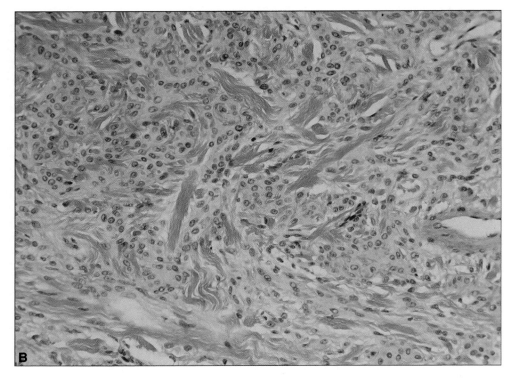

Histologically, hamartomas are composed of varying proportions of adipose and fibroglandular tissue, usually with a circumscribed border (Figure 7.4A). The ducts and lobules are histologically unremarkable and the stroma is generally paucicellular and fibrotic with admixed adipose tissue (Figure 7.4B). A unique

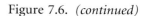
Figure 7.6. *(continued)*

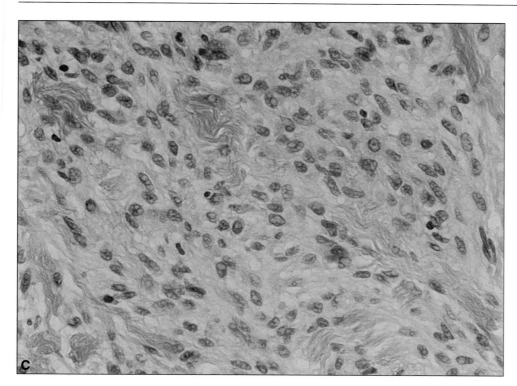

variant contains a prominent smooth muscle proliferation within the stroma; these lesions are referred to as myoid hamartoma (Figures 7.5A,B). There is no prognostic significance attributed to this distinction.

Hamartomas are benign lesions and complete excision is the treatment of choice. Additional therapy is not recommended and to date there have been no reports of recurrences.

MYOFIBROBLASTOMA

Myofibroblastomas are uncommon lesions that can occur in men and women and usually present as a palpable mass. Breast imaging generally reveals a circumscribed, lobulated mass that is devoid of calcifications.

Microscopically, myofibroblastomas are composed of a circumscribed proliferation of bland, spindled cells that are haphazardly arranged amongst bands of hyalinized collagen (Figure 7.6A). The constituent cells have round to oval nuclei without significant nuclear pleomorphism or mitotic activity (Figures 7.6B,C). These tumors are typically positive for desmin, actin, and CD34 and negative for keratins. The differential diagnosis includes fibromatosis, nodular fasciitis, spindle cell carcinoma, and solitary fibrous tumor. Fibromatosis generally has an infiltrative border and the component cells do not stain with CD34 but will frequently express β-catenin (see subsequent section). Nodular fasciitis has a characteristic loosely cellular appearance with associated inflammation and extravasated red blood cells (Figure 7.7). Spindle cell carcinoma (metaplastic carcinoma) generally has more nuclear pleomorphism and mitotic activity; keratin immunohistochemistry can aid in this distinction (Figures 7.8A,B). There is histologic and immunohistochemical

Figure 7.7. Nodular fasciitis. Unlike myofibroblastoma, these tumors are loosely cellular with associated inflammation and extravasated red blood cells.

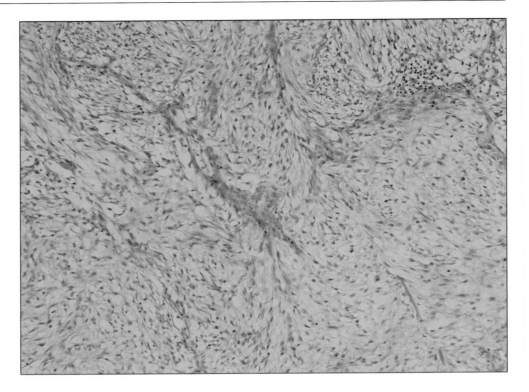

Figures 7.8. (A,B) Spindle cell carcinoma (metaplastic carcinoma). Unlike myofibroblastoma, these tumors typically have more significant nuclear pleomorphism and mitotic activity. In difficult cases, keratin immunohisto-chemistry will highlight the epithelial nature of these tumors; myofibroblastomas are negative for cytokeratin.

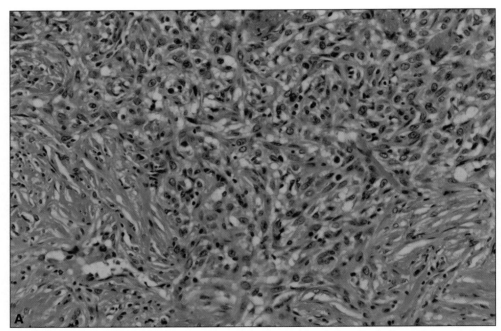

overlap between myofibroblastoma and solitary fibrous tumor and although some authors suggest differentiating these tumors, we feel they are likely within the same spectrum of myofibroblastic proliferations and do not make this distinction.

Treatment for myofibroblastoma is complete surgical excision. Recurrences have not been reported.

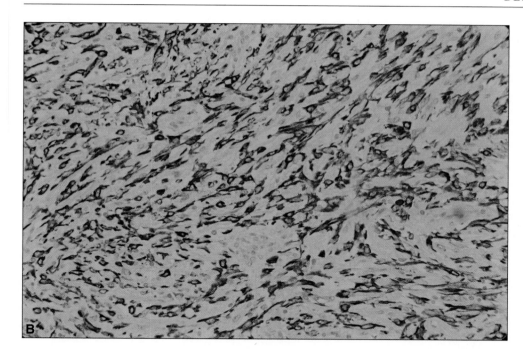

Figure 7.8. *(continued)*

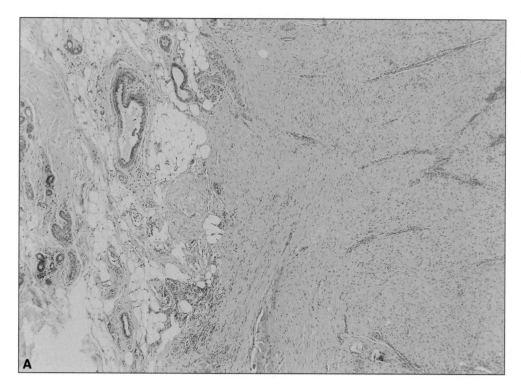

Figure 7.9. (A) Fibromatosis. Spindle cell proliferation with infiltrative border compatible with mammary fibromatosis.

FIBROMATOSIS

Fibromatosis is an uncommon lesion in the breast that usually presents as a painless mass. Imaging often shows a stellate mass that can mimic a

Figure 7.9. *(continued)* (B,C) Fibromatosis. Higher power showing the spindle cells characteristic of fibromatosis. The cells are oval to spindled with little pleomorphism or mitotic activity.

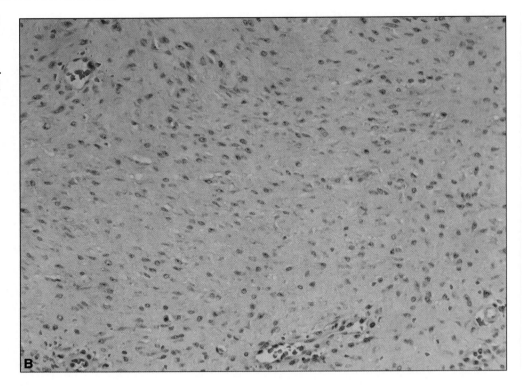

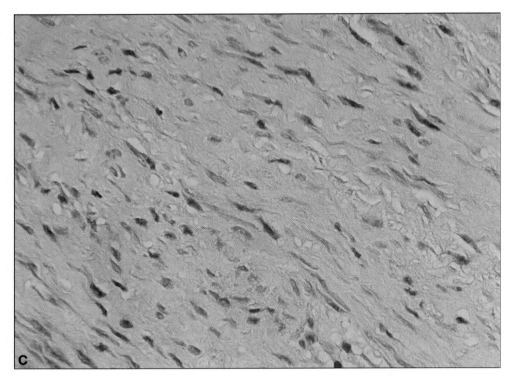

carcinoma. Fibromatosis can occur at any age and has been described in men and women.

Microscopically, mammary fibromatosis is an infiltrative process composed of bland spindle cells and is identical to that seen in other organs

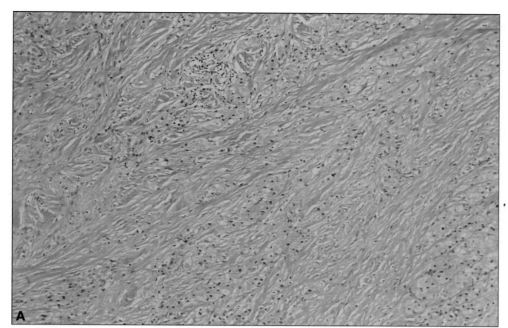

Figure 7.10. (A) Granular cell tumor. Sheets and cords of pale cells with abundant eosinophilic cytoplasm appear to infiltrate within a collagenous stroma.
(B) Granular cell tumor. Higher power of the tumor in A showing the cytology characteristic of this tumor. The cells are round to polygonal with abundant eosinophilic cytoplasm and bland nuclei.

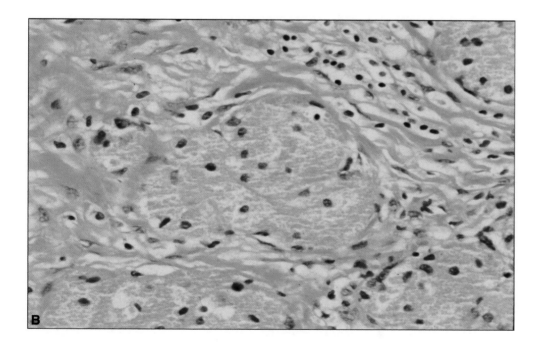

(Figure 7.9A). The constituent cells are oval to spindled without significant pleomorphism (Figures 7.9B,C). Mitotic activity can be seen but should not exceed 3/10 hpfs. Immunohistochemistry for β-catenin can be particularly useful as a significant percentage of cases show nuclear positivity. The differential diagnosis is similar to that of myofibroblastoma (see prior section).

The treatment is complete surgical excision with attention paid to clear margins. Recurrences are more common in lesions that are inadequately excised. There are no reports of metastases although these tumors can be locally aggressive due to their infiltrative nature.

GRANULAR CELL TUMOR

Granular cell tumor of the breast is rare and has been reported in both men and women. Typically, patients present with a solitary mass. Imaging is nonspecific and can show a circumscribed or infiltrative mass lesion.

Microscopically, granular cell tumors of the breast are histologically similar in appearance to those occurring in other organs (Figure 7.10A). The tumors are composed of sheets of cells with abundant granular, eosinophilic cytoplasm although sometimes the cytoplasm can appear clear or vacuolated (Figure 7.10B). Nuclei are generally small but some nuclear pleomorphism is acceptable. Mitotic activity is rare. The periphery of the lesion is frequently infiltrative. The cells of granular cell tumor are PAS-positive/diastase-resistant and stain positive for S-100 and vimentin. Carcinoembryonic antigen (CEA) can also be positive but variably. The cells are negative for cytokeratins.

Treatment consists of excision with clear margins. Recurrences have been reported in the literature. Rarely, cases of malignant granular cell tumor have been reported. Histologic features that are worrisome include marked pleomorphism, necrosis, and increased mitotic activity; however, these features are not specific for a diagnosis of malignant granular cell tumor as a report of supposed metastatic granular cell tumor had a benign-appearing primary.

REFERENCES

Abraham, S. C., C. Reynolds, et al. (2002). "Fibromatosis of the breast and mutations involving the APC/beta-catenin pathway." *Hum Pathol* 33(1): 39–46.

Adeniran, A., H. Al-Ahmadie, et al. (2004). "Granular cell tumor of the breast: a series of 17 cases and review of the literature." *Breast J* 10(6): 528–31.

Adwani, A., N. Bees, et al. (2006). "Hemangioma of the breast: clinical, mammographic, and ultrasound features." *Breast J* 12(3): 271.

Boulat, J., M. P. Mathoulin, et al. (1994). "[Granular cell tumors of the breast]." *Ann Pathol* 14(2): 93–100.

Brodie, C. and E. Provenzano (2008). "Vascular proliferations of the breast." *Histopathology* 52(1): 30–44.

Charpin, C., M. P. Mathoulin, et al. (1994). "Reappraisal of breast hamartomas. A morphological study of 41 cases." *Pathol Res Pract* 190(4): 362–71.

Chiacchio, R., L. Panico, et al. (1999). "Mammary hamartomas: an immunohistochemical study of ten cases." *Pathol Res Pract* 195(4): 231–6.

Cohen, M. A., E. A. Morris, et al. (1996). "Pseudoangiomatous stromal hyperplasia: mammographic, sonographic, and clinical patterns." *Radiology* 198(1): 117–20.

Damiani, S., R. Dina, et al. (1999). "Eosinophilic and granular cell tumors of the breast." *Semin Diagn Pathol* 16(2): 117–25.

Daroca, P. J., Jr., R.J. Reed, et al. (1985). "Myoid hamartomas of the breast." *Hum Pathol* 16(3): 212–9.

Devouassoux-Shisheboran, M., M. D. Schammel, et al. (2000). "Fibromatosis of the breast: age-correlated morphofunctional features of 33 cases." *Arch Pathol Lab Med* 124(2): 276–80.

Dunne, B., A. H. Lee, et al. (2003). "An immunohistochemical study of metaplastic spindle cell carcinoma, phyllodes tumor and fibromatosis of the breast." *Hum Pathol* 34(10): 1009–15.

Ferreira, M., C. T. Albarracin, et al. (2008). "Pseudoangiomatous stromal hyperplasia tumor: a clinical, radiologic and pathologic study of 26 cases." *Mod Pathol* 21(2): 201–7.

Fisher, C. J., A. M. Hanby, et al. (1992). "Mammary hamartoma – a review of 35 cases." *Histopathology* 20(2): 99–106.

Gocht, A., H. C. Bosmuller, et al. (1999). "Breast tumors with myofibroblastic differentiation: clinico-pathological observations in myofibroblastoma and myofibrosarcoma." *Pathol Res Pract* 195(1): 1–10.

Ibrahim, R. E., C. G. Sciotto, et al. (1989). "Pseudoangiomatous hyperplasia of mammary stroma. Some observations regarding its clinicopathologic spectrum." *Cancer* 63(6): 1154–60.

Lee, A. H. (2008). "Recent developments in the histological diagnosis of spindle cell carcinoma, fibromatosis and phyllodes tumour of the breast." *Histopathology* 52(1): 45–57.

Meguerditchian, A. N., D. A. Malik, et al. (2008). "Solitary fibrous tumor of the breast and mammary myofibroblastoma: the same lesion?" *Breast J* 14(3): 287–92.

Mercado, C. L., S. A. Naidrich, et al. (2004). "Pseudoangiomatous stromal hyperplasia of the breast: sonographic features with histopathologic correlation." *Breast J* 10(5): 427–32.

Murugesan, J. R., S. Joglekar, et al. (2006). "Myoid hamartoma of the breast: case report and review of the literature." *Clin Breast Cancer* 7(4): 345–6.

Oberman, H. A. (1989). "Hamartomas and hamartoma variants of the breast." *Semin Diagn Pathol* 6(2): 135–45.

Polger, M. R., C. M. Denison, et al. (1996). "Pseudoangiomatous stromal hyperplasia: mammographic and sonographic appearances." *AJR Am J Roentgenol* 166(2): 349–52.

Powell, C. M., M. L. Cranor, et al. (1995). "Pseudoangiomatous stromal hyperplasia (PASH). A mammary stromal tumor with myofibroblastic differentiation." *Am J Surg Pathol* 19(3): 270–7.

Rosen, P. P. and D. Ernsberger (1989). "Mammary fibromatosis. A benign spindle-cell tumor with significant risk for local recurrence." *Cancer* 63(7): 1363–9.

Rosen, P. P. and R. L. Ridolfi (1977). "The perilobular hemangioma. A benign microscopic vascular lesion of the breast." *Am J Clin Pathol* 68(1): 21–3.

Salomao, D. R., T. B. Crotty, et al. (2001). "Myofibroblastoma and solitary fibrous tumour of the breast: histopathologic and immunohistochemical studies." *Breast* 10(1): 49–54.

Stafyla, V., N. Kotsifopoulos, et al. (2007). "Myoid hamartoma of the breast: a case report and review of the literature." *Breast J* 13(1): 85–7.

Vos, L. D., A. T. R. T. Tjon, et al. (1994). "Granular cell tumor of the breast: mammographic and histologic correlation." *Eur J Radiol* 19(1): 56–9.

Vuitch, M. F., P. P. Rosen, et al. (1986). "Pseudoangiomatous hyperplasia of mammary stroma." *Hum Pathol* 17(2): 185–91.

Wargotz, E. S., H. J. Norris, et al. (1987). "Fibromatosis of the breast. A clinical and pathological study of 28 cases." *Am J Surg Pathol* 11(1): 38–45.

Wargotz, E. S., S. W. Weiss, et al. (1987). "Myofibroblastoma of the breast. Sixteen cases of a distinctive benign mesenchymal tumor." *Am J Surg Pathol* 11(7): 493–502.

8 LOBULAR NEOPLASIA (NONINVASIVE)

Geza Acs, MD, PhD

Clinical Features	95
Macroscopic and Microscopic Features	96
Differential Diagnosis	108
Treatment and Prognosis	118

The term lobular carcinoma in situ (LCIS) was introduced by Foote and Stewart in 1941. They described this characteristic proliferation within breast lobules and recognized its cytologic similarity and frequent association with invasive lobular carcinoma. In subsequent years, morphologically similar but less well-developed lesions were termed atypical lobular hyperplasia (ALH), although various authors used different criteria to distinguish them from LCIS. Acknowledging the fact that distinction of LCIS and ALH depends solely on the extent of the proliferation, the term lobular neoplasia (LN) was suggested to encompass the full range of proliferations. The concept of lobular intraepithelial neoplasia (LIN) was also proposed and suggested, grading these lesions based on the extent of proliferation and cytologic features (LIN 1-3); however, it did not gain wide acceptance in clinical practice. Recently, variant forms of LCIS have also been described including lesions with central comedo-type necrosis and ones with high-grade cytologic features (termed pleomorphic LCIS [PLCIS]). Despite similar morphology, maintaining the distinction between LCIS and ALH appears to have a clinical significance as ALH is associated with a lower risk of development of subsequent carcinoma when formal criteria are used for their distinction. In the subsequent discussion of LCIS and ALH, the term LN will be used as an inclusive term for both entities.

CLINICAL FEATURES

LCIS and ALH have no specific clinical or radiologic features and they are usually diagnosed as incidental findings in breast biopsies performed for other reasons. Although their true incidence in the general population is not known, LCIS and ALH are relatively uncommon lesions identified in 1–3.6 percent of breast biopsies. The incidence of LN is greatest before the menopause with an average age at diagnosis of 44–46 years; less than 10 percent of patients are postmenopausal. LN tends to be multicentric in the same breast in about 50 percent of the cases and bilateral in a little more than one-third of the cases when the contralateral breast is biopsied. LN tends to involve the breast in greatest extent in the areas containing the most breast parenchyma, including the central area beneath the nipple and the upper outer quadrant. Although usually no mass is associated with LN, the proliferations may involve other benign breast lesions that can present as clinical masses or architectural distortion on mammography, such as fibroadenomas, sclerosing adenosis, or radial scars. Although LN is usually not associated with microcalcifications except in cases when it involves benign lesions containing them, calcifications in adjacent benign breast tissue is often present. Indeed, some studies suggest that LN may be present in up to 10 percent of breast biopsies targeting mammographic microcalcifications. In contrast to usual LN, variant forms (PLCIS) may present with features similar to high-grade ductal carcinoma in situ (DCIS), either as a mass or with pleomorphic mammographic calcifications, especially when central comedo-type necrosis is present.

MACROSCOPIC AND MICROSCOPIC FEATURES

LCIS and ALH are not associated with any specific gross findings.

Microscopically, LN in its classic form is characterized by a dyscohesive proliferation of evenly spaced, uniform, small cuboidal cells with moderate amounts of light or clear cytoplasm. The nuclei are uniform, bland, round to oval with absent or inconspicuous nucleoli (Figure 8.1). The nuclei are often eccentrically placed giving the cells a plasmacytoid appearance. Mitotic figures are rare, but occasionally may be present. The constituent cells often contain intracytoplasmic vacuoles containing mucin (Figure 8.2), which can be highlighted with periodic acid Schiff (PAS) or mucicarmine stains. Occasionally, these intracytoplasmic vacuoles are large enough to give the cells a signet-ring appearance (Figure 8.3). In contrast to these classic (or "type A") cytologic features, other LN lesions are characterized by neoplastic cells with more abundant cytoplasm, larger nuclei with more variation in size and shape and conspicuous nucleoli (Figure 8.4). These latter examples are referred to as "type B" LN. In occasional cases, proliferations may contain a mixture of type A and B cells.

As mentioned, LCIS and ALH are composed of similar cells and the main distinction between these lesions is based on the extent of involvement of breast lobules. Although diagnostic criteria used by different authors vary, the most widely accepted and clinically validated criteria are those described by Page and coworkers. According to these criteria, the diagnosis of LCIS requires that the involved spaces are occupied by a uniform population of characteristic neoplastic cells and that these cells completely fill and distend at least 50 percent of the acini within the involved lobular units (Figure 8.5). For practical purposes, full distension of acini as required for a diagnosis of LCIS means eight or more neoplastic cells across the diameter of the acinus. In cases when less than 50 percent of the acini are filled and expanded, the filling of the acini is incomplete with residual intercellular spaces present or other cell types are intermixed with the neoplastic cells, ALH is diagnosed (Figures 8.6 and 8.7).

Although LN usually involves the lobules, the characteristic neoplastic cells may also involve larger ducts, usually in a so-called "pagetoid" fashion. In these cases the

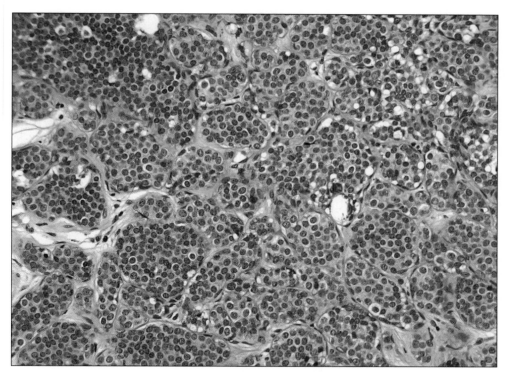

Figure 8.1. Both lobular carcinoma in situ (LCIS) and atypical lobular hyperplasia (ALH) are composed of a proliferation of similar characteristic neoplastic cells. The constituent cells are small, uniform with regular, round nuclei without nucleoli, and scant amounts of light or clear cytoplasm.

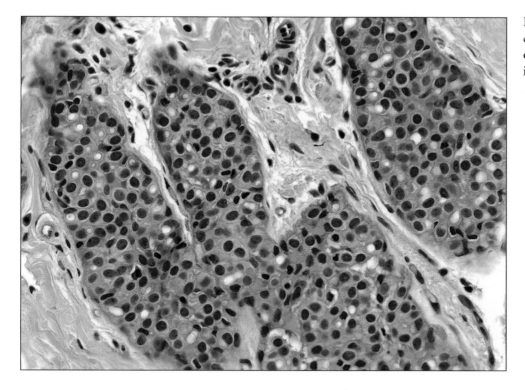

Figure 8.2. The constituent cells of lobular neoplasia often contain small intracytoplasmic vacuoles.

characteristic cells of LN undermine the normal luminal epithelial lining cells and insinuate themselves either singly or in small groups between the luminal cells and the myoepithelial layer of the ducts (Figure 8.8). In postmenopausal women with atrophic lobules, involvement of small ducts may be the only manifestation of LN.

Figure 8.3. The intracytoplasmic vacuoles in some cases of lobular neoplasia may be large and prominent and produce a signet-ring cell appearance.

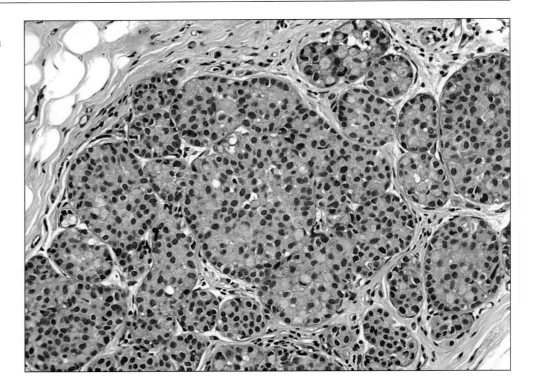

Figure 8.4. "Type B" or large-cell lobular neoplasia composed of dyscohesive neoplastic cells with more abundant cytoplasm, larger nuclei, and sometimes conspicuous nucleoli.

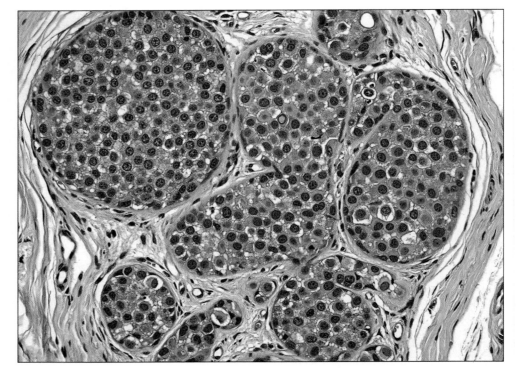

In these cases, the affected small ducts have been described as resembling a clover leaf (Figure 8.9). When LCIS is present, pagetoid ductal involvement does not affect risk implication. In contrast, when such an involvement is associated with ALH, the subsequent risk of carcinoma was reported to be intermediate between those of

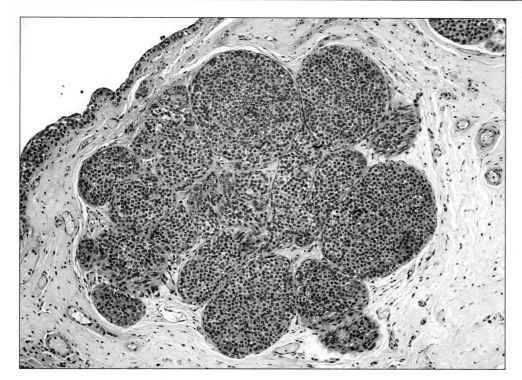

Figure 8.5. Lobular carcinoma in situ (LCIS). Virtually all acini in this lobule are completely filled and distended by a uniform population of the characteristic neoplastic cells.

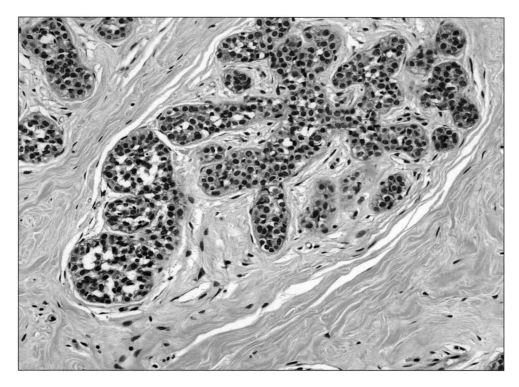

Figure 8.6. Atypical lobular hyperplasia (ALH). Although some of the acini are completely filled, they are not expanded and residual intercellular spaces are present. A second population of cells with small, dark, pyknotic appearing nuclei is also seen.

ALH and LCIS alone. Difficulty arises in some cases when only pagetoid involvement of ducts with characteristic cells is identified in a biopsy without the typical proliferations occupying the lobules. Although pagetoid involvement of ducts is more common in cases of LCIS compared to ALH, in such cases a diagnosis of

Figure 8.7. Atypical lobular hyperplasia (ALH). Although the acini are filled and expanded, the characteristic cells of lobular neoplasia are admixed with those of usual hyperplasia.

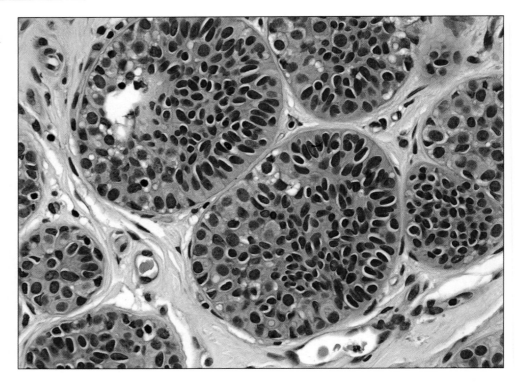

Figure 8.8. Ductal involvement by cells of lobular neoplasia. The characteristic neoplastic cells undermine the normal luminal lining cells and insinuate themselves between the luminal and myoepithelial cells in a "pagetoid" fashion.

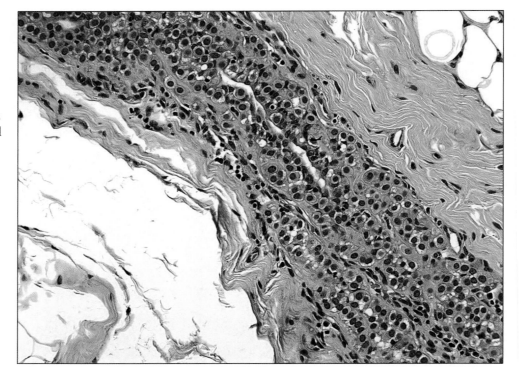

ductal involvement by cells of LN can be made. The risk implications of these lesions without well-defined ALH or LCIS are not clear.

LN may sometimes involve otherwise benign lesions, such as florid usual hyperplasia, sclerosing adenosis, radial scars, intraductal papillomas, fibroadenomas, or

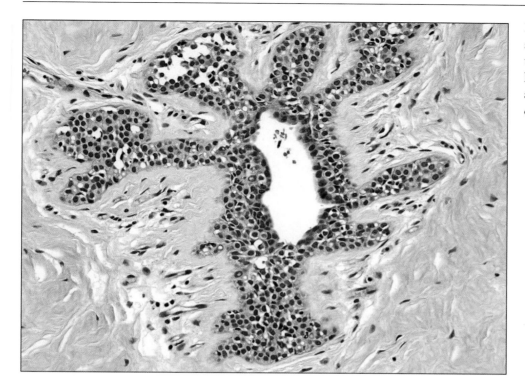

Figure 8.9. Involvement of a small duct may sometimes be the only manifestation of lobular neoplasia. The affected duct resembles a clover leaf.

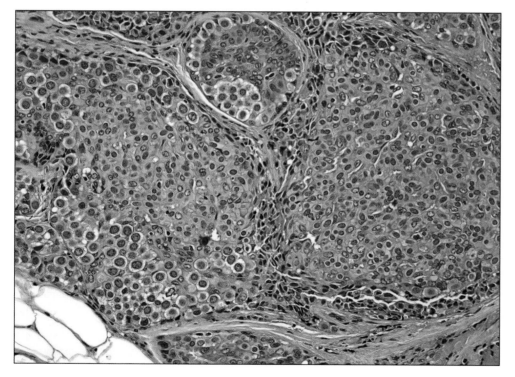

Figure 8.10. Lobular neoplasia involving florid usual hyperplasia. Occasionally, the residual spaces present in usual hyperplasia together with the monotypic cell population of lobular neoplasia may mimic ductal carcinoma in situ.

collagenous spherulosis (Figures 8.10 through 8.15), raising the differential diagnosis of either invasive or in situ ductal carcinoma (see Differential Diagnosis).

A characteristic molecular alteration in LN is the absence of membrane expression of the epithelial adhesion molecule E-cadherin. The lack of this expression

Figure 8.11. Lobular neoplasia involving sclerosing adenosis. The presence of a monotypic cell population within the distorted spaces of sclerosing adenosis may mimic invasive carcinoma. Recognition of the maintenance of a lobulocentric architecture in sclerosing adenosis at low power and the presence of myoepithelial cells are clues to the correct diagnosis.

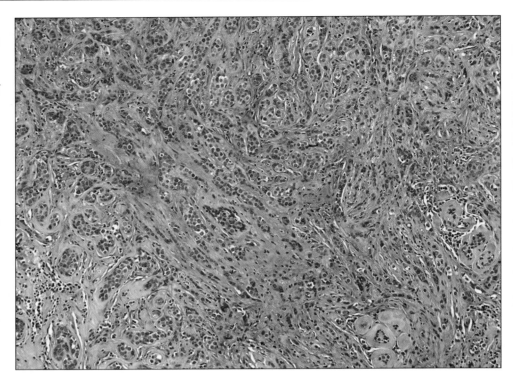

Figure 8.12. Lobular neoplasia involving radial scar. The sclerosis and distortion in radial scars and the presence of the monotypic neoplastic cells of lobular neoplasia may mimic invasive carcinoma.

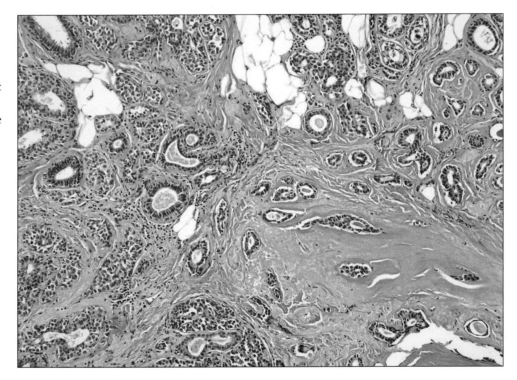

may be due to mutations of the E-cadherin gene (CDH1) located at 16q22.1, loss of heterozygosity (LOH) at 16q22, or the methylation of the promoter of the E-cadherin gene. The resulting loss of E-cadherin protein expression can be detected by immunohistochemistry in cases of LN (Figure 8.16). The vast majority

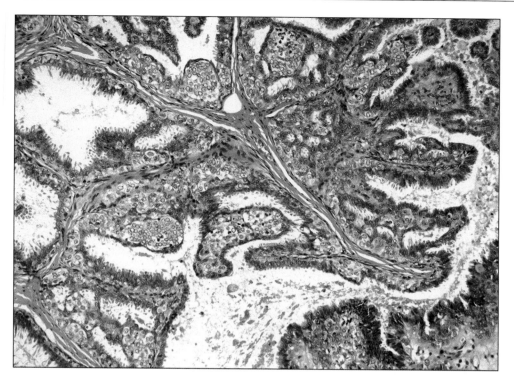

Figure 8.13. Lobular neoplasia involving intraductal papilloma. The neoplastic cells insinuate themselves between the lining epithelial cells of the papillae and the myoepithelial cell layer.

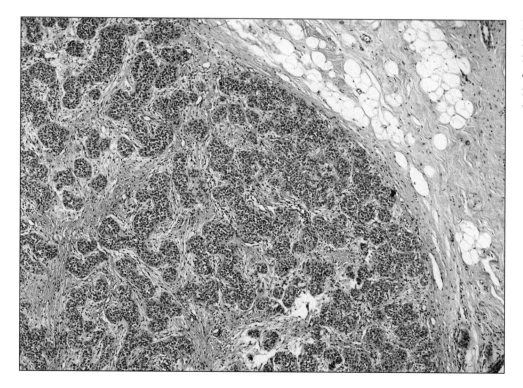

Figure 8.14. Lobular neoplasia involving fibroadenoma. The characteristic neoplastic cells fill the epithelial spaces within the lesion.

of these cases show complete loss of E-cadherin membrane expression in contrast with benign breast elements and DCIS, which uniformly express this protein in their cell membranes. LN and invasive lobular carcinomas also show characteristic cytoplasmic staining with p120 catenin, in contrast to its membrane staining

Figure 8.15. Lobular neoplasia involving collagenous spherulosis. Although the lesion contains a uniform population of neoplastic cells and appears fenestrated, the lumens of collagenous spherulosis contain a fibrillar material and are lined by a layer of myoepithelial cells.

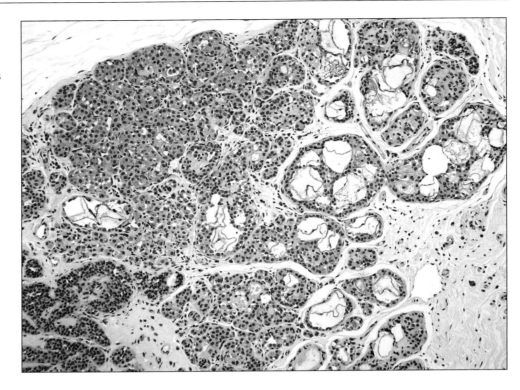

Figure 8.16. The cells of lobular neoplasia show a characteristic loss of membrane expression of E-cadherin by immunohistochemistry. Note that focal staining may be seen in myoepithelial cells and occasional residual normal epithelial cells.

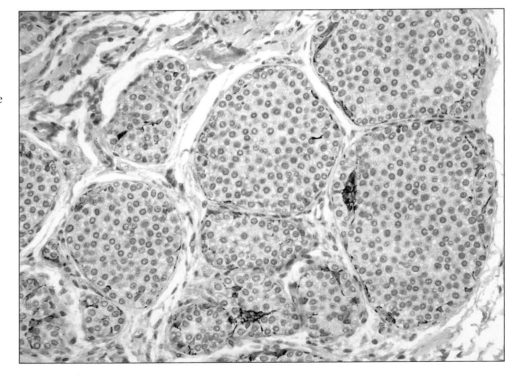

pattern in ductal lesions. A recent study has suggested that immunohistochemistry for high-molecular-weight cytokeratins using the 34betaE12 antibody is positive in LN and negative in DCIS, however, more recent studies have shown more equivocal results.

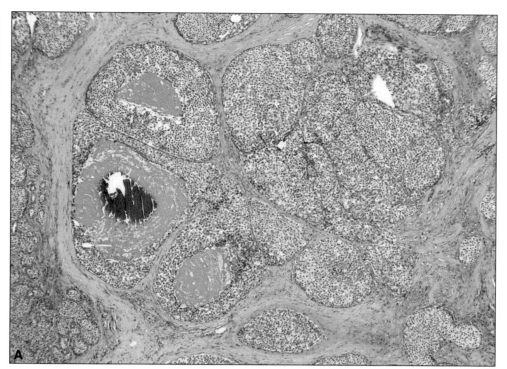

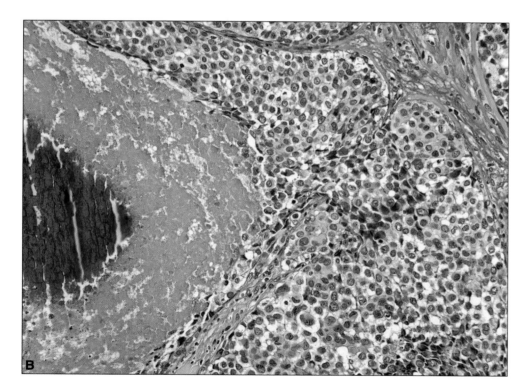

Figure 8.17. Lobular carcinoma in situ with central comedo-type necrosis and calcification. (A) The proliferation of uniform characteristic neoplastic cells greatly expands lobules and ducts and may form clinical mass lesions. (B) Despite the presence of necrosis, the constituent cells are uniform without high-grade cytologic features, similar to cells of usual type B lobular neoplasia. Mitotic figures are unapparent.

In recent years, several variant forms of LN have been described, including LCIS with comedo-type necrosis, pleomorphic LCIS, and LN with signet-ring cell or apocrine features. LCIS with comedo-type necrosis is characterized by a prolifer-ation of dyscohesive neoplastic cells similar to usual LCIS, but the lesions show

Figure 8.17. *(continued)*
(C) Immunohistochemistry
shows complete loss of
membrane reactivity for
E-cadherin in the constituent
neoplastic cells.

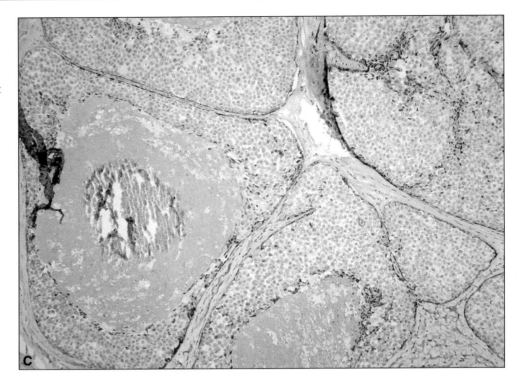

prominent extension of lobules and even larger ducts with central areas of comedo-type necrosis (Figure 8.17). Some authorities regard this variant as an extreme form of ductal involvement by LCIS. PLCIS is composed of neoplastic cells showing the characteristic dyscohesive growth pattern of LN, but they show distinctly larger nuclei with marked pleomorphism, prominent nucleoli and increased presence of mitotic figures (Figure 8.18). Some cases of PLCIS show prominent apocrine differentiation (Figure 8.19). Although signet-ring cells may be seen in many benign and malignant breast lesions, LCIS with high-grade cytologic features are often associated with the presence of prominent signet-ring cells (Figure 8.20) Central necrosis and calcifications, similar to those seen in high-grade DCIS, may be present, and occasionally these proliferations may form clinical mass lesions. In such cases, usual LN is frequently present in the surrounding breast tissue. In rare cases, cells similar to those of PLCIS show proliferations of a lesser extent that do not fulfill formal criteria for LCIS or only involve other benign breast lesions in a pagetoid fashion (Figure 8.21). Although it is not established clearly in the literature, similar to the case of atypical ductal proliferations where high-grade cytology excludes the diagnosis of atypical ductal hyperplasia and places the lesion in the category of DCIS, LN with high-grade nuclear features should be diagnosed as PLCIS regardless of the extent of the proliferation. Of note, invasive lobular carcinoma, either pleomorphic or usual, is present in the majority of cases of PLCIS.

Cells of LN, including PLCIS, are positive for estrogen receptor (ER) and progesterone receptor (PR) expression in 90–100 percent of the cases. Usual LN is uniformly negative for HER2/neu overexpression, but a small percentage (4 percent) of PLCIS may be HER2/neu positive. In keeping with the relatively

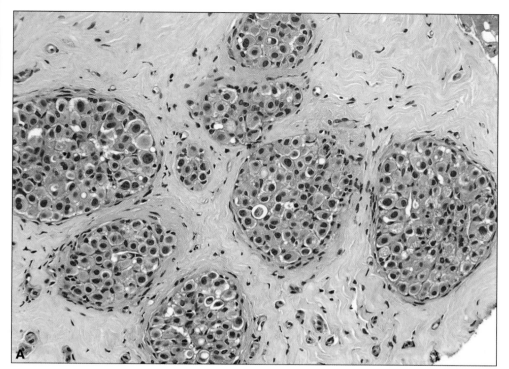

Figure 8.18. Pleomorphic lobular carcinoma in situ. (A) These lesions are composed of neoplastic cells showing the characteristic dyscohesive growth pattern of lobular neoplasia, but they show distinctly larger nuclei with marked pleomorphism. (B) The constituent cells show high-grade cytologic features with prominent and often multiple nucleoli.

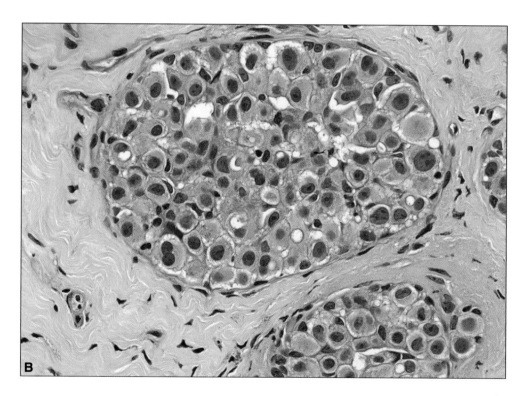

frequent presence of mitotic figures in PLCIS, studies have shown an increased proliferation rate in these lesions compared to usual LN using Ki-67 immunohistochemistry and also have suggested a higher rate of aberrant p53 expression.

Figure 8.18. *(continued)* (C) The constituent cells of pleomorphic lobular carcinoma in situ show complete loss of E-cadherin membrane expression.

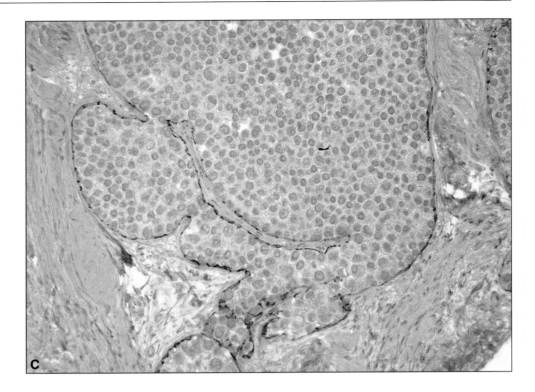

Figure 8.19. Pleomorphic lobular carcinoma in situ with apocrine features.

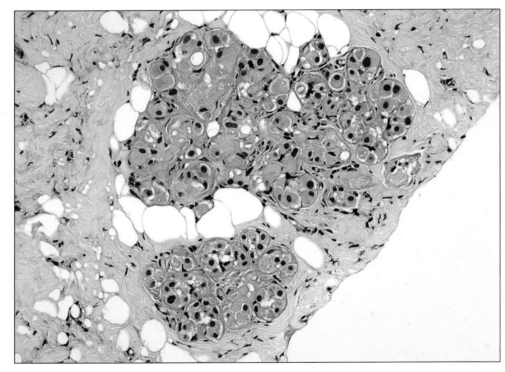

DIFFERENTIAL DIAGNOSIS

With regard to differential diagnosis it is important to emphasize that the diagnosis of LN is based on the characteristic dyscohesive growth pattern and cytologic

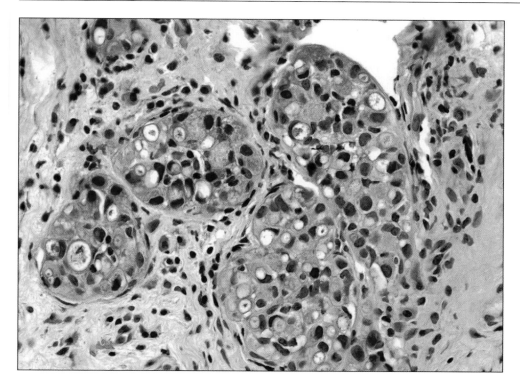

Figure 8.20. Pleomorphic lobular carcinoma in situ with signet-ring cell features.

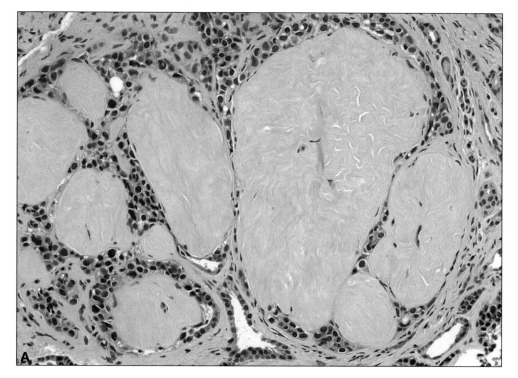

Figure 8.21. Pleomorphic lobular carcinoma in situ involving a small fibroadenoma. (A) Although there is only limited proliferation of the characteristic cells within the lesion, the presence of high grade cytologic features warrants a diagnosis of lobular carcinoma in situ.

features of the constituent neoplastic cells irrespective of their location in the ductal or lobular system of the breast. In rare cases, the differentiation of LCIS from DCIS may pose difficulties, however, it is important because of its therapeutic implications. This distinction is most difficult in cases of solid pattern low-grade DCIS

Figure 8.21. *(continued)*
(B) The neoplastic cells of
pleomorphic lobular
carcinoma are negative for
E-cadherin expression.

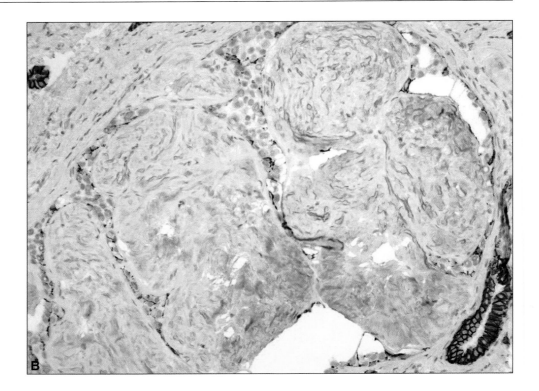

Figure 8.22. Low-grade solid
ductal carcinoma in situ
(DCIS). In solid pattern
ductal carcinoma in situ, the
neoplastic cells appear
cohesive and in most cases, at
least focally, form small
secondary spaces or
microacini with the
surrounding cells polarized
toward the small lumens.

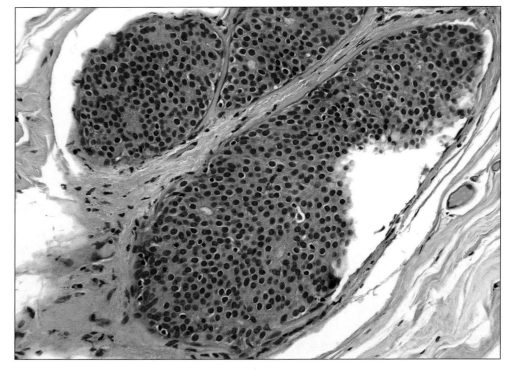

involving acini (termed "cancerization of lobules") with little or no lobular distortion. In solid pattern DCIS the neoplastic cells in most cases, at least focally, form
small secondary spaces or microacini with the surrounding cells polarized toward
the small lumens (Figure 8.22). The cells of LN tend to be dyscohesive with rounded

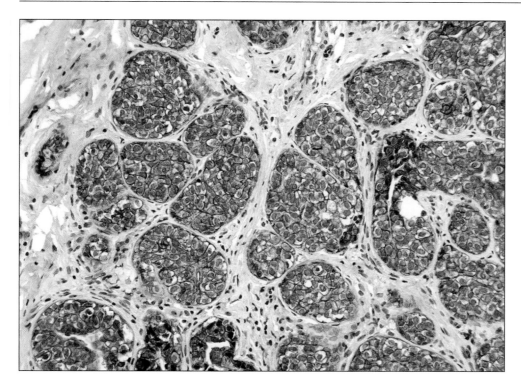

Figure 8.23. Low-grade solid ductal carcinoma in situ shows diffuse, strong membrane expression of E-cadherin by immunohistochemistry.

cytoplasm detached from one another, in contrast with the cohesive, sharply circumscribed, crisp cell membranes of DCIS. In contrast to DCIS, intracytoplasmic vacuoles are frequently present in LCIS. The cells of DCIS tend to show polarization toward the myoepithelial cells and basement membrane, a feature not found in LCIS. E-cadherin immunostaining is helpful in most cases, with the cells of LCIS being negative and those of DCIS showing positive membrane staining (Figure 8.23).

Diagnostic difficulty may occur in occasional cases when poor tissue fixation leads to the appearance of dyscohesive cells within a lobule (Figure 8.24). Prominent myoepithelial cells may also be confused with the cells of LN, particularly when the latter involve extralobular ducts in a pagetoid fashion. In contrast to LN cells, myoepithelial cells tend to have small, dark nuclei, clear indiscernible cytoplasm, and lack the characteristic dyscohesive appearance of LN cells. Immunohistochemical stains for myoepithelial markers may be useful in rare challenging cases.

Partial involvement by LN of benign lesions such as collagenous spherulosis and usual hyperplasia may mimic the appearance of cribriform spaces amongst a proliferation of uniform cells mimicking cribriform DCIS. The involvement of usual hyperplasia with single cells of LN may mimic atypical ductal proliferations due to the uniform population of neoplastic cells and the presence of secondary spaces. One has to recognize the distinct cytologic features of the individual LN cells with round nuclei and relatively abundant clear or light cytoplasm in these cases. E-cadherin immunostaining is often of limited use in these cases as the absent membrane immunoreactivity of the single LN cells is masked by the positive membrane staining of the surrounding benign epithelial cells and one should look for small clusters of LN cells within the lesions with absent membrane staining within the clusters (Figure 8.25). The involvement of collagenous spherulosis may pose a particular challenge. Although at low power both cribriform DCIS and collagenous

Figure 8.24. Poor tissue fixation may lead to the appearance of dyscohesive cells within a lobule mimicking lobular neoplasia.

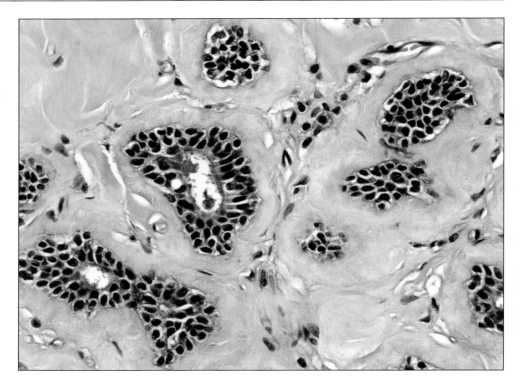

Figure 8.25. Lobular neoplasia involving usual hyperplasia. The absent E-cadherin membrane immunoreactivity of the single lobular neoplasia cells can be masked by the positive membrane staining of the surrounding benign epithelial cells.

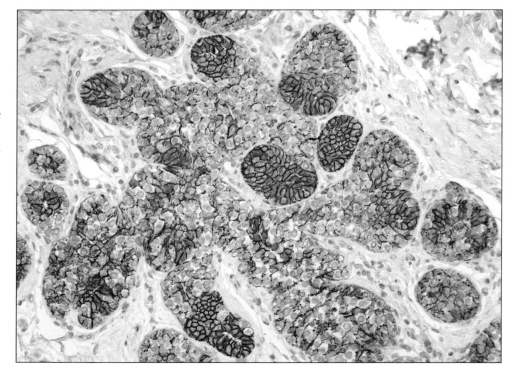

spherulosis involved by LN contain a uniform population of neoplastic cells and appear fenestrated, the lumens of collagenous spherulosis contain characteristic eosinophilic spherules composed of hyaline of fibrillar material as opposed to the lumens of cribriform DCIS, which tend to be empty or contain necrotic material

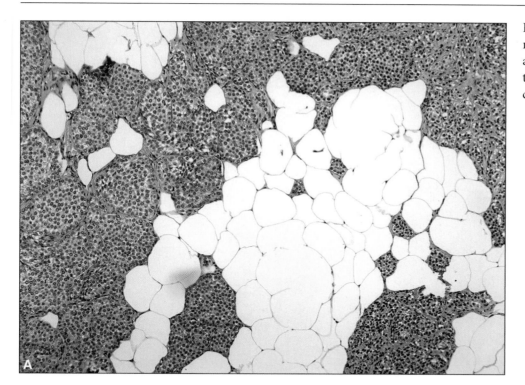

Figure 8.26. (A) Lobular neoplasia involving irregular adenosis within adipose tissue mimicking invasive carcinoma.

and calcifications in some cases. In addition, the spherules of collagenous spherulosis are lined by a layer of myoepithelial cells, which can be highlighted by immunohistochemical stains for myoepithalial markers. Immunostains for E-cadherin are also useful in this situation.

LN rarely involves otherwise benign breast lesions that may present as a clinically detectable mass. Sclerosing adenosis, fibroadenomas, or intraductal papillomas may contain foci of LN. On occasion, involvement of complex sclerosing lesions and sclerosing adenosis by LN may mimic invasive carcinoma. Recognition of the underlying architecture of these benign proliferations and the characteristic cytologic features of LN cells within the lesions provide a key to the correct diagnosis. Since the underlying benign lesions are characterized by maintenance of a myoepithelial-cell layer, immunohistochemistry for myoepithelial markers, such as p63 and smooth muscle myosin heavy chain, can be useful in difficult cases. LN involving microglandular, tubular, or irregular adenosis may appear to infiltrate breast parenchyma and adipose tissue in a haphazard fashion and can mimic invasive carcinoma (Figure 8.26). Recognition of the underlying architecture including residual glands not involved by LN, together with demonstration of a myoepithelial layer by immunohistochemistry, help establish the correct diagnosis.

PLCIS and LCIS with comedo-type necrosis can also present diagnostic difficulties in addition to therapeutic dilemmas (see Treatment and Prognosis). Since the cytologic features of PLCIS are similar to those of high-grade DCIS, distinction may be particularly challenging if the proliferations form mass lesions, and necrosis and calcifications are present. In addition, DCIS may occasionally appear dyshesive due to either single-cell necrosis and/or tissue fixation (Figure 8.27). Since all PLCIS cases reported to date have been negative for E-cadherin by immunohistochemistry, immunohistochemical stains for this marker are useful in this distinction. In fact,

Figure 8.26. *(continued)*
(B) Immunohistochemistry for myoepithelial markers (e.g., calponin) highlights the myoepithelial cells.
(C) Lobular neoplasia involving extensive tubular adenosis mimicking invasive carcinoma.
(D) Immunohistochemical stains for calponin highlight the presence of myoepithelial cells.

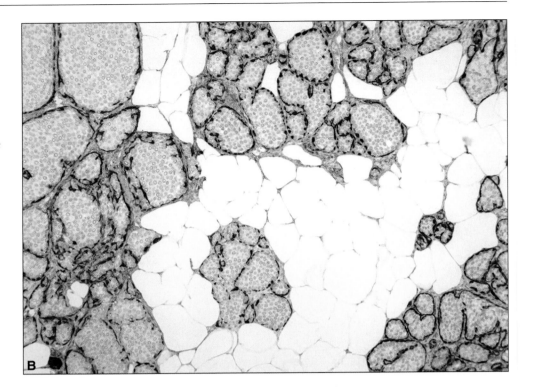

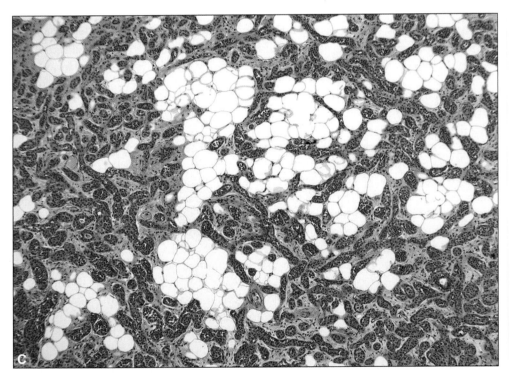

most authorities would not diagnose a lesion as PLCIS if it shows membranous E-cadherin reactivity.

Although some in-situ carcinomas clearly have features of both LCIS and DCIS on routine histology, it must be kept in mind that these diagnoses are not mutually

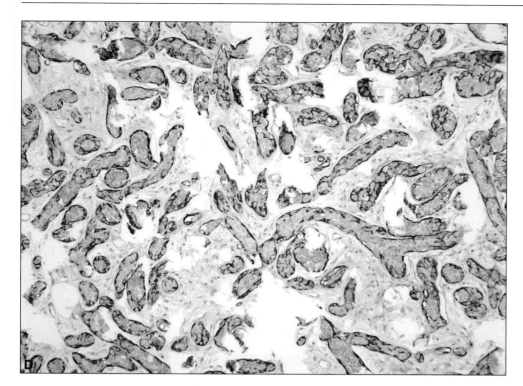

Figure 8.26. *(continued)*

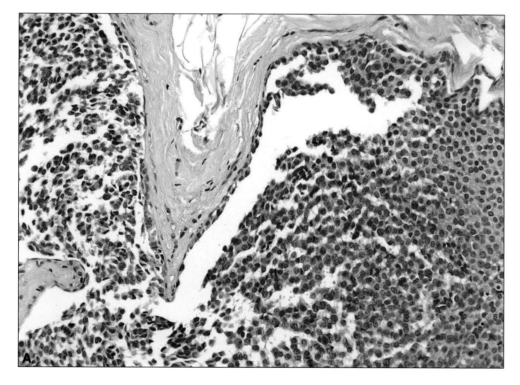

Figure 8.27. (A) Solid ductal carcinoma in situ with "pseudodyshesion" due to poor fixation may mimic lobular carcinoma in situ.

exclusive. LCIS and DCIS may coexist in the same breast and even in the same terminal duct-lobular units (Figure 8.28). When classic features of both LN and DCIS in distinct components of the lesions involving the same spaces are present, a diagnosis of in-situ carcinoma, mixed ductal and lobular type can be rendered. The

Figure 8.27. *(continued)*
(B) E-cadherin
immunohistochemistry
shows strong membrane
expression in the cells of solid
ductal carcinoma in situ.

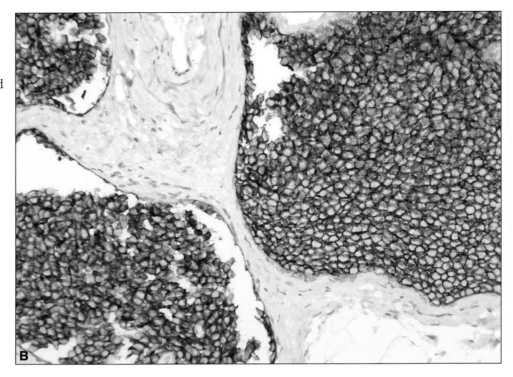

Figure 8.28 (A,B) Mixed
in-situ carcinoma with clearly
distinct components of ductal
carcinoma in situ and lobular
carcinoma in situ present in
the same spaces. (C) An
E-cadherin stain highlights
the distinct lobular and ductal
components.

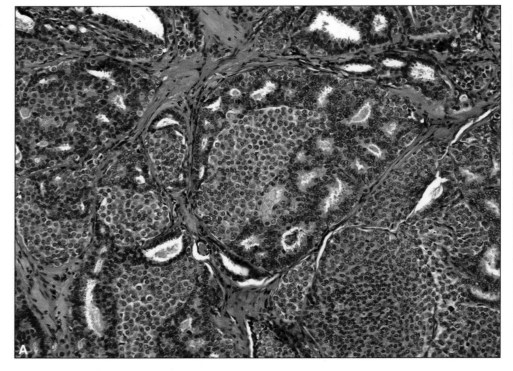

distinct ductal and lobular components of these mixed lesions can usually be highlighted by E-cadherin immunostaining. The distinct components often show differential hormone receptor and HER2/neu expression as well, especially when the
DCIS component is high grade.

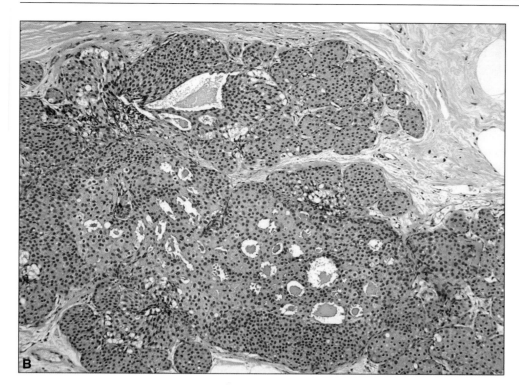

Figure 8.28. *(continued)*

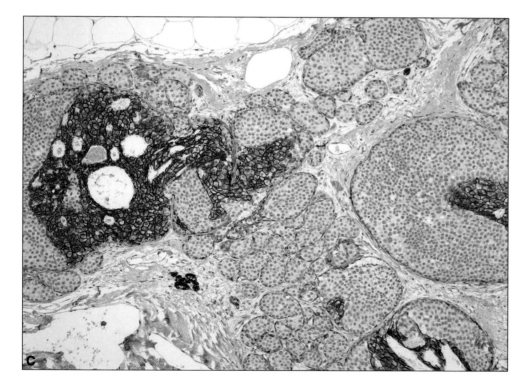

Finally, some in-situ carcinomas display features of both LCIS and DCIS making categorization difficult if not impossible on routine histology. Approximately, two-thirds of these lesions will show absent or diffuse strong membrane E-cadherin reactivity supporting their classification as LCIS or DCIS, respectively. In about one-third of these cases, however, the constituent cells show a mixture of E-cadherin-negative and -positive immunoreactivity, suggesting that they may represent cases of in-situ carcinoma with a truly mixed ductal and lobular phenotype.

TREATMENT AND PROGNOSIS

When Foote and Steward first described LCIS, they considered this lesion a precursor for invasive lobular carcinoma and recommended mastectomy for treatment. Subsequent studies indicated that although LCIS is associated with an increased risk of later development of carcinoma, this risk is relatively small. Furthermore, the carcinomas detected could occur in both breasts and showed either lobular or ductal (no special type) histology. Based on these observations, LCIS was generally regarded a risk indicator rather than a true precursor for invasive carcinoma, conferring increased risk for the development of carcinoma in either breast. Compared to control populations the relative risk of subsequent cancer after a diagnosis of LCIS is in the range between 7 and 11. In terms of absolute risk, patients with a diagnosis of LCIS have a 1–2 percent risk of developing carcinoma per year and a lifetime risk of 30–40 percent. The time taken for the development of cancer from an initial biopsy with LCIS is relatively long ranging from 15 to 30 years in the various studies; however, it appears to be highest in the first 15 years. Some studies also suggest that the risk is decreased after the menopause. Studies that separated ALH from LCIS lesions indicated that the risk associated with ALH is approximately half of that associated with LCIS (4–5 times vs. 7–11 times). Separation of ALH from LCIS based on strict criteria thus can help in risk stratification and patient management and justifies their distinction in clinical practice. The risk associated with PLCIS and LCIS with necrosis is unclear, but it is thought to be higher than that for classic LCIS.

The risk of development of carcinoma after a diagnosis of LN is bilateral and it used to be a common belief that this risk was equal for both breasts. More recent studies, however, demonstrated that the development of carcinoma is three times more likely in the ipsilateral compared to the contralateral breast, closely reflecting the rate of bilaterality of LN. Indeed, in studies where the contralateral breast was also biopsied and found to be negative for the presence of LN, the development of carcinoma in the contralateral breast was very low. Although both invasive lobular or ductal (no special type) carcinoma may develop in patients with LN, the frequency of invasive lobular carcinoma in these cases is much higher compared to patients without LN or the general population. Recent molecular studies also revealed the presence of similar genetic alterations, including similar mutations in the E-cadherin (CDH1) gene in invasive lobular carcinoma and associated LCIS. Thus, the morphologic and immunophenotypic similarity of LN and invasive lobular carcinoma, the preferential development of ipsilateral carcinomas with lobular histology after a diagnosis of LN, the occasional presence of microinvasive lobular carcinoma associated with LN, and the presence of similar molecular alterations in these lesions all support the view that ALH and LCIS can act as true precursor lesions for invasive lobular carcinoma, in addition to being risk indicators. At the present time, however, no histologic or molecular features have been identified to predict which LN lesions may act as direct precursors. Although both ALH and LCIS lack E-cadherin expression by immunohistochemistry and often show LOH at 16q22, recent studies have suggested that mutations in the CDH1 gene only occur in LCIS cases and it was suggested that this molecular feature may represent a step toward the development of invasive carcinoma.

In contrast to DCIS, which is considered to be a precursor lesion to invasive carcinoma, the clinical approach to patients with LCIS and ALH is still largely based on the belief that they mainly represent a generalized risk factor and these patients are managed conservatively with careful observation and the addition of selective ER modulators, such as tamoxifen. This clinical management also implies that reporting on the margin status for LN is not necessary. In light of the recent observations indicating that LN is a unilateral predictor of breast cancer risk and a likely direct precursor to invasive carcinoma, it was suggested that surgical intervention removing most of the glandular tissue of the breast may markedly reduce the risk of carcinoma in these patients while preserving cosmesis. This approach however, has not yet been validated in clinical trials or accepted in clinical management.

Variant forms of LCIS, such as PLCIS and LCIS with comedo-type necrosis, present challenging difficulties in management. Given the relative rarity of these lesions, our current knowledge of their biologic behavior, ipsilateral or contralateral risk implications, and natural history is limited. A few studies and anecdotal reports suggest that these cases are more frequently associated with invasive carcinoma compared to usual LCIS and ALH. The study of Sneige and coworkers, although limited by short follow-up, suggests that complete excision in these cases is important. In the absence of large studies with clinical outcome data, at the present time we recommend complete excision of these lesions similar to the management of DCIS. Since these variant lesions are associated with usual LN in most cases, surgical management should focus on the complete removal of the variant lesion in cases when breast conservation is preferred. Rare, histologically indeterminate lesions with a mixture of E-cadherin negative and positive cells should probably be managed similarly.

Given the widespread use of core needle biopsy (CNB) for the initial evaluation of mammographically detected breast lesions, the identification of LN on CNB has become more frequent and presents particular difficulties in management. Given the frequent multifocality and bilaterality of LN, if these lesions are accepted primarily as markers of generalized increased risk for the development of carcinoma, it seems logical to conclude that excision is not necessary when LN is an incidental finding and the additional histologic findings in the biopsy (i.e., microcalcifications in benign lesions or fibroadenoma) account for the mammographic lesions targeted by the biopsy. On the other hand, several studies examining the risk of carcinoma on follow-up surgical excision after a diagnosis of LN on CNB found that carcinoma was identified in an average of 16 and 26 percent of the cases with a CNB diagnosis of ALH and LCIS, respectively. However, it should be kept in mind that all these studies included a relatively small number of cases and were retrospective with inherent bias in cases with regard to surgical excision. In agreement with others, we believe that it is most prudent to utilize a multidisciplinary approach in these cases with clinical, radiological, and pathologic correlation. We currently recommend excision for patients when the histologic findings do not correlate with the mammographic features of the targeted lesion or another high-risk lesion, such as atypical ductal hyperplasia, is also present in the CNB, which requires excision irrespective of the presence of LN. Given the higher likelihood of the presence of invasive carcinoma associated with PLCIS or LCIS with comedo-type necrosis, surgical excision is indicated when these lesions are identified on CNB.

REFERENCES

Acs G, Lawton TJ, Rebbeck TR, et al. Differential expression of E-cadherin in lobular and ductal neoplasms of the breast and its biologic and diagnostic implications. *Am J Clin Pathol.* 2001;115:85–98.

Berx G, Cleton-Jansen AM, Strumane K, et al. E-cadherin is inactivated in a majority of invasive human lobular breast cancers by truncation mutations throughout its extracellular domain. *Oncogene.* 1996;13:1919–25.

Berx G, van RF. The E-cadherin/catenin complex: an important gatekeeper in breast cancer tumorigenesis and malignant progression. *Breast Cancer Res.* 2001;3:289–93.

de Leeuw WJ, Berx G, Vos CB, et al. Simultaneous loss of E-cadherin and catenins in invasive lobular breast cancer and lobular carcinoma in situ. *J Pathol.* 1997;183:404–11.

Dupont WD, Page DL. Risk factors for breast cancer in women with proliferative breast disease. *N Engl J Med.* 1985;312:146–51.

Fadare O, Dadmanesh F, Varado-Cabrero I, et al. Lobular intraepithelial neoplasia [lobular carcinoma in situ] with comedo-type necrosis: a clinicopathologic study of 18 cases. *Am J Surg Pathol.* 2006;30:1445–53.

Jacobs TW, Connolly JL, Schnitt SJ. Nonmalignant lesions in breast core needle biopsies: to excise or not to excise? *Am J Surg Pathol.* 2002;26:1095–110.

Jacobs TW, Pliss N, Kouria G, et al. Carcinomas in situ of the breast with indeterminate features: role of E-cadherin staining in categorization. *Am J Surg Pathol.* 2001;25: 229–36.

Lakhani SR, Audretsch W, Cleton-Jensen AM, et al. The management of lobular carcinoma in situ (LCIS). Is LCIS the same as ductal carcinoma in situ (DCIS)? *Eur J Cancer.* 2006;42:2205–11.

Liberman L, Sama M, Susnik B, et al. Lobular carcinoma in situ at percutaneous breast biopsy: surgical biopsy findings. *AJR Am J Roentgenol.* 1999;173:291–9.

Marshall LM, Hunter DJ, Connolly JL, et al. Risk of breast cancer associated with atypical hyperplasia of lobular and ductal types. *Cancer Epidemiol Biomarkers Prev.* 1997;6:297–301.

Mastracci TL, Tjan S, Bane AL, et al. E-cadherin alterations in atypical lobular hyperplasia and lobular carcinoma in situ of the breast. *Mod Pathol.* 2005;18:741–51.

Middleton LP, Grant S, Stephens T, et al. Lobular carcinoma in situ diagnosed by core needle biopsy: when should it be excised? *Mod Pathol.* 2003;16:120–9.

Page DL, Dupont WD, Rogers LW. Ductal involvement by cells of atypical lobular hyperplasia in the breast: a long-term follow-up study of cancer risk. *Hum Pathol.* 1988;19:201–7.

Page DL, Dupont WD, Rogers LW, et al. Atypical hyperplastic lesions of the female breast: A long-term follow-up study. *Cancer.* 1985;55:2698–708.

Page DL, Schuyler PA, Dupont WD, et al. Atypical lobular hyperplasia as a unilateral predictor Rosen PP, Braun DW, Jr., Lyngholm B, et al. Lobular carcinoma in situ of the breast: preliminary results of treatment by ipsilateral mastectomy and contralateral breast biopsy. *Cancer.* 1981;47:813–19.of breast cancer risk: a retrospective cohort study. *Lancet.* 2003;361:125-9.

Rosen PP, Braun DW, Jr., Lyngholm B, et al. Lobular carcinoma in situ of the breast: preliminary results of treatment by ipsilateral mastectomy and contralateral breast biopsy. *Cancer.* 1981;47:813–19.

Rosen PP, Kosloff C, Lieberman PH, et al. Lobular carcinoma in situ of the breast. Detailed analysis of 99 patients with average follow-up of 24 years. *Am J Surg Pathol.* 1978;2:225–51.

Schnitt SJ, Morrow M. Lobular carcinoma in situ: current concepts and controversies. *Semin Diagn Pathol.* 1999;16:209–23.

Sneige N, Wang J, Baker BA, et al. Clinical, histopathologic, and biologic features of pleomorphic lobular (ductal-lobular) carcinoma in situ of the breast: a report of 24 cases. *Mod Pathol.* 2002;15:1044–50.

Vos CB, Cleton-Jansen AM, Berx G, et al. E-cadherin inactivation in lobular carcinoma in situ of the breast: an early event in tumorigenesis. *Br J Cancer.* 1997;76:1131–3.

Wheeler JE, Enterline HT, Roseman JM, et al. Lobular carcinoma in situ of the breast. Long-term followup. *Cancer.* 1974;34:554–63.

9 DUCTAL NEOPLASIA

Beiyun Chen, MD, PhD

Ductal Hyperplasia and Atypical Ductal Hyperplasia	122
Ductal Carcinoma in situ	124
Flat Epithelial Atypia	133

Intraductal proliferative lesions are a group of cytologically and architecturally diverse proliferations, typically originating from the terminal duct-lobular unit (TDLU) and confined to the mammary duct lobular system. They are traditionally divided into three broad categories: usual ductal hyperplasia (UDH), atypical ductal hyperplasia (ADH), and ductal carcinoma in situ (DCIS), and are associated with different levels of risk for subsequent development of invasive breast cancer, ranging from approximately 1.5–2 times that of the reference population for UDH, to 4–5-fold for ADH, and 8–10-fold for DCIS. The entity flat epithelial atypia (FEA) will also be illustrated in this chapter.

DUCTAL HYPERPLASIA AND ATYPICAL DUCTAL HYPERPLASIA

UDH is a benign ductal proliferative lesion typically characterized by irregularly shaped and sized secondary lumens, often peripherally distributed, and streaming of the central proliferating cells. Epithelial bridges are thin and stretched; nuclei are unevenly distributed. Cytologically, the lesion is composed of cells with indistinct cell borders and variation in the shape and size of the nuclei. An admixture of epithelial, myoepithelial, or metaplastic apocrine cells is not uncommon (Figures 9.1–9.3).

ADH is defined as an intraductal proliferative lesion that has "some, but not all, the features of low-grade ductal carcinoma in situ." In practice, this distinction can be quite difficult as evidenced by several interobserver variability studies on intraductal proliferative lesions (see References). Thus, in making this diagnosis, it is critical to understand the criteria for the diagnosis of low-grade DCIS, which will be discussed later. In general, we reserve this diagnosis for cases in which either the architecture is that of low-grade DCIS (generally a micropapillary or cribriform pattern) but the cell population is not monomorphic, or the cells involved are a

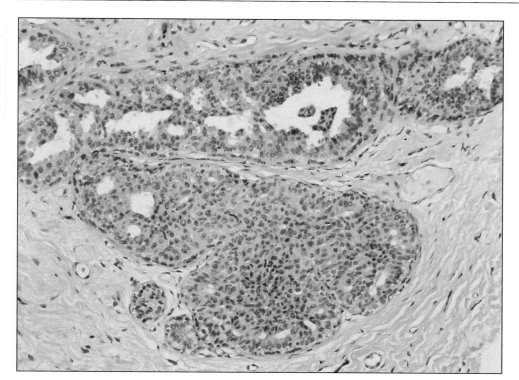

Figure 9.1. Intraductal proliferation forming irregular fenestrations and stretched epithelial bridges.

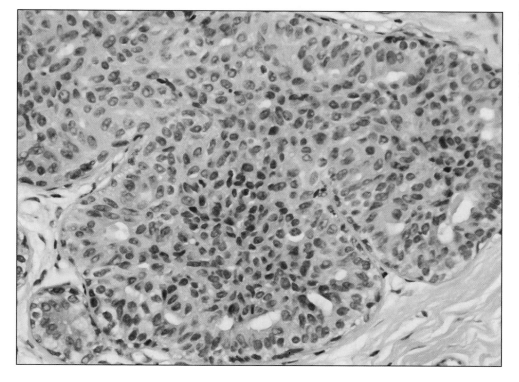

Figure 9.2. Solid intraductal proliferation of a heterogeneous cell population with overlapping nuclei and peripheral fenestrations.

monomorphic population but the architecture falls short of that seen in low-grade DCIS (Figures 9.4 and 9.5). In addition, quantitative criteria can be used when a case that fulfills criteria for low-grade DCIS is only focally present either in a single duct or the focus measures less than 0.2 cm.

Figure 9.3. Heterogeneous population of cells, haphazardly arranged, forming irregularly shaped secondary lumens.

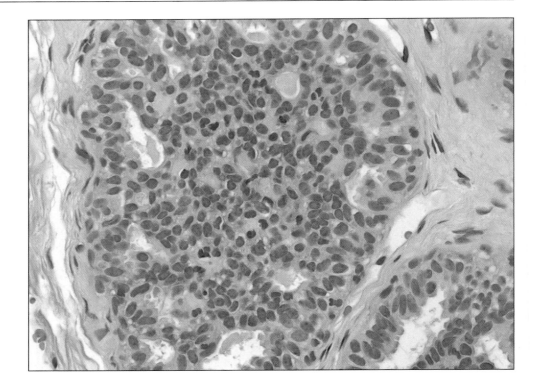

Figure 9.4. Ductal proliferation of relatively monomorphic cells forming arcades and fronds in a micropapillary/cribriform pattern; however, note the "tapering" of the micropapillae and incomplete involvement of the duct spaces.

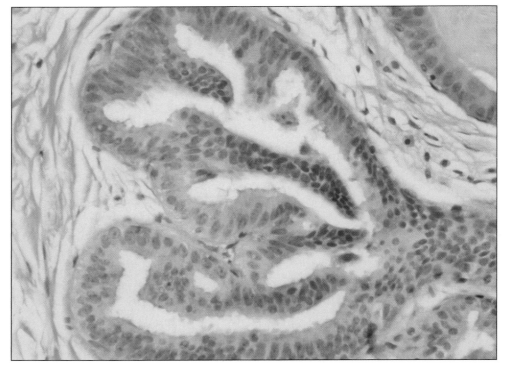

DUCTAL CARCINOMA IN SITU

DCIS is a heterogeneous group of neoplastic intraductal lesions characterized by increased epithelial proliferation of different architectural patterns and various

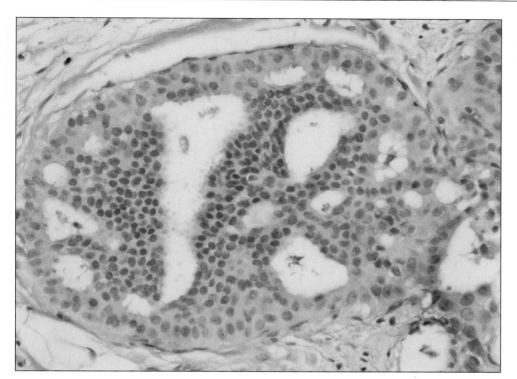

Figure 9.5. A similar proliferation of relatively monomorphic cells in a cribriform pattern but with irregular secondary lumen formation.

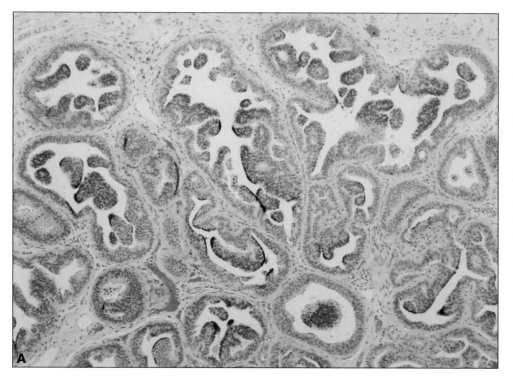

Figure 9.6. (A–C) Low-grade micropapillary ductal carcinoma in situ. The proliferation occupies numerous duct spaces and is composed of a monotonous population of low-grade nuclei growing in a micropapillary pattern. Focally, some "roman bridge" pattern is seen, which is typical as micropapillary and cribriform patterns often coexist.

degrees of cytological atypia ranging from mild to severe. DCIS is generally divided into three categories based on nuclear grade. The architectural patterns typically encountered are micropapillary, cribriform, solid, and papillary. Within any lesion, however, a mix of nuclear grade and architectural types can be seen.

Figure 9.6. *(continued)*

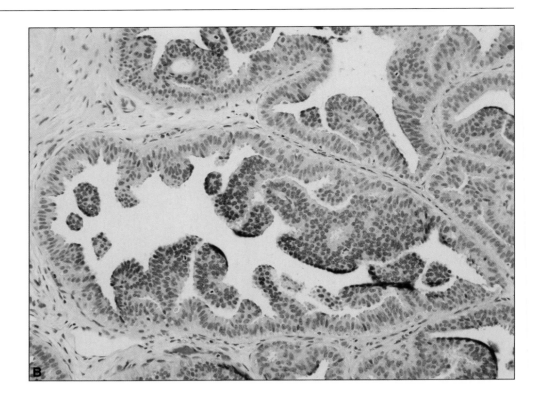

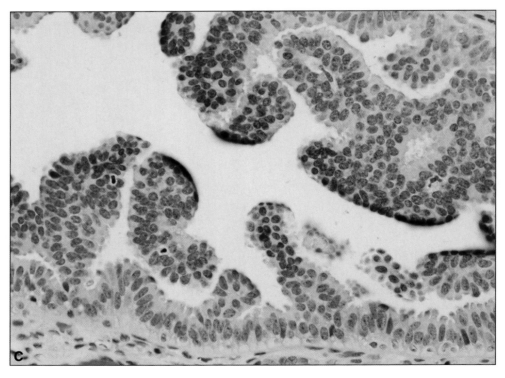

Low-grade DCIS is composed of small, monomorphic cells, growing in arcades, micropapillae, cribriform or solid patterns (Figures 9.6A–C and 9.7–9.9). The nuclei are uniform in size and have a regular chromatin pattern with inconspicuous nuclei. Mitotic figures are rare. The minimal extent of involvement for a diagnosis

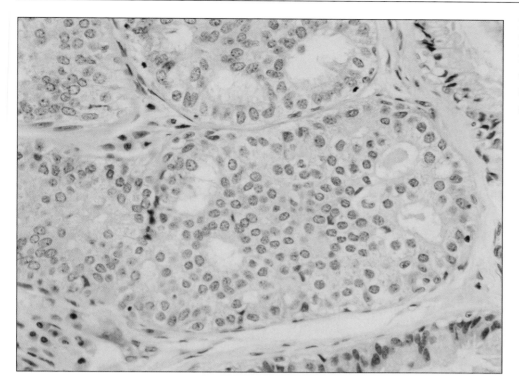

Figures 9.7. Cribriform low-grade DCIS. The cytology is low grade and the cells are oriented around architecturally rigid secondary lumens.

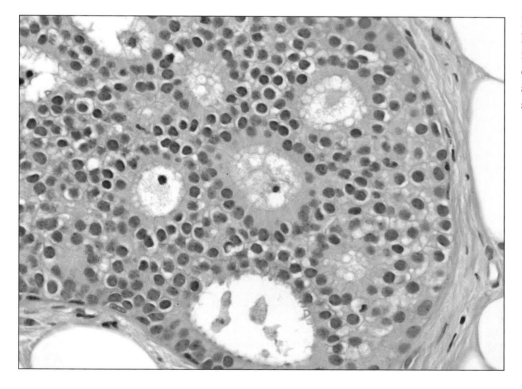

Figures 9.8. Cribriform low-grade DCIS. The cytology is low grade and the cells are oriented around architecturally rigid secondary lumens.

of low-grade DCIS includes complete involvement of a single-duct cross-section, two spaces, or one or more duct cross-sections of greater than 2 mm in diameter. As mentioned, if a process of fulfilling the cytologic and architectural criteria falls short, a diagnosis of ADH should be made.

Figure 9.9. Solid low-grade DCIS. Note the monotypic population of low-grade cells with inconspicuous nucleoli.

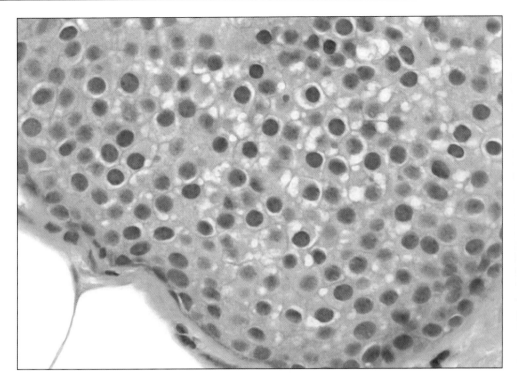

Figure 9.10. (A,B) High-grade DCIS with central necrosis. Note the high-grade cytology with marked nuclear pleomorphism and prominent nucleoli.

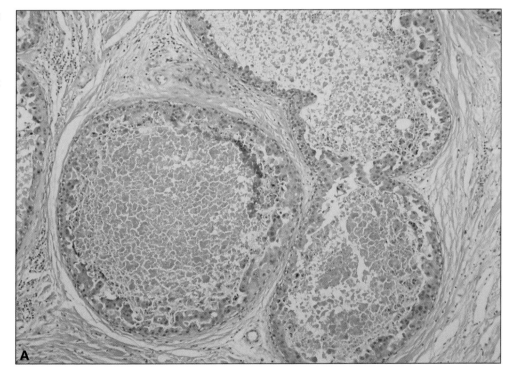

On the contrary, high-grade DCIS is composed of markedly atypical cells proliferating within ducts, although the growth patterns can be similar to low-grade DCIS. The nuclei of high-grade DCIS are very pleomorphic, poorly polarized, with irregular contour and distribution with coarse, clumped chromatin and prominent

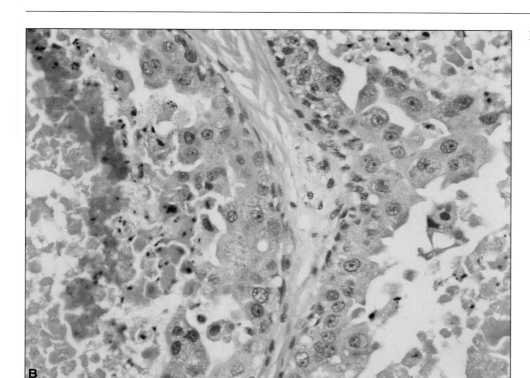

Figure 9.10. *(continued)*

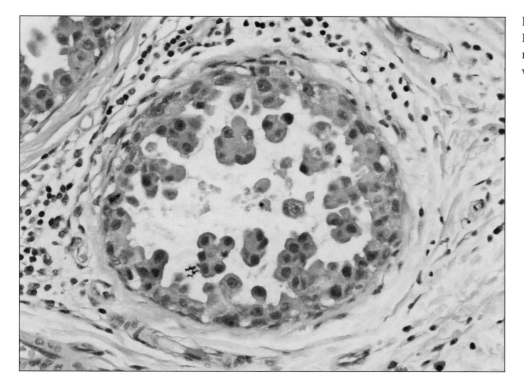

Figure 9.11. High-grade DCIS growing in a micropapillary pattern without central necrosis.

nucleoli. Central necrosis is very common but not obligatory (Figures 9.10A,B and 9.11). Unlike in low-grade DCIS, even a single layer of highly anaplastic cells lining the duct in a flat fashion or a single <1 mm duct with the typical morphologic features is sufficient for this diagnosis (Figure 9.12).

Figure 9.12. High-grade DCIS. Although the cells appear to only be a single layer lining the duct spaces, there is marked nuclear pleomorphism and mitotic activity.

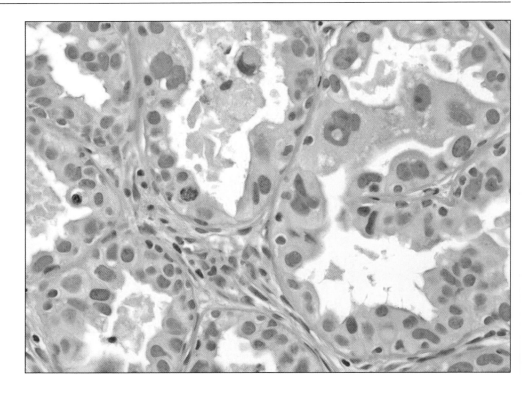

Figure 9.13. Solid DCIS with intermediate nuclear grade. Nucleoli are identifiable at low power. Necrosis is focally present in the involved duct at the upper left.

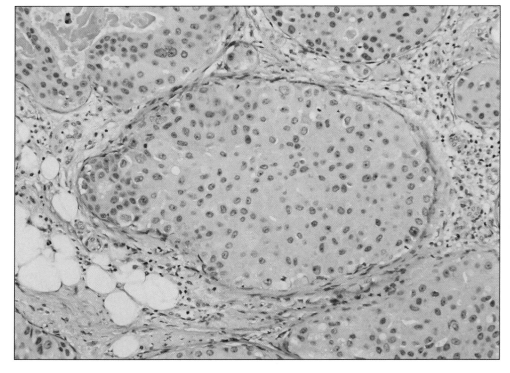

The category of intermediate grade DCIS was developed for those cases in which the cells were not as pleomorphic as high-grade DCIS but exhibited more cytology atypia and less low-grade monotony than that seen in low-grade DCIS (Figure 9.13). Necrosis can also be seen more commonly in intermediate-grade

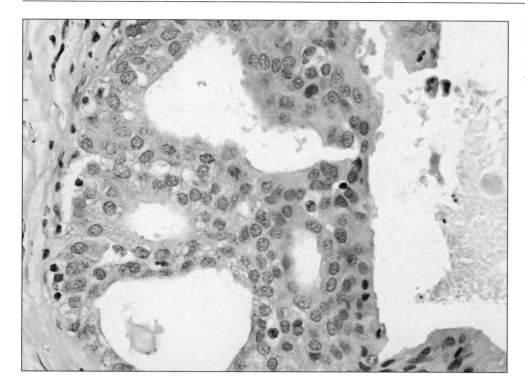

Figure 9.14. Cribriform DCIS with intermediate nuclear grade and focal central necrosis.

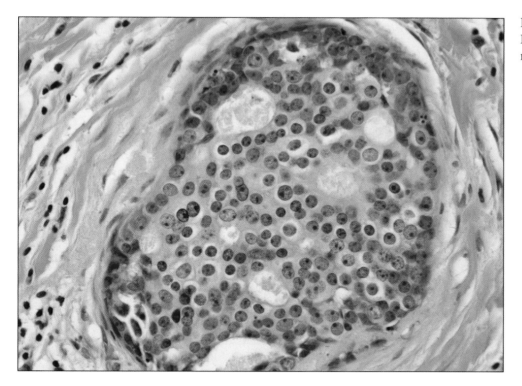

Figure 9.15. Cribriform DCIS with intermediate nuclear grade.

DCIS (Figure 9.14). The architectural growth patterns are similar to the other nuclear grades (Figure 9.15).

All forms of DCIS can extend into surrounding lobules (so-called cancerization of lobules), although this tends to be more common in high-grade DCIS. Often

Figure 9.16. (A,B) High-grade DCIS with microinvasion. Although there is cancerization of lobules and abundant sclerosis that distorts the architecture, there are a few small clusters of cells appearing outside the lobular unit that meet the criteria for microinvasion.

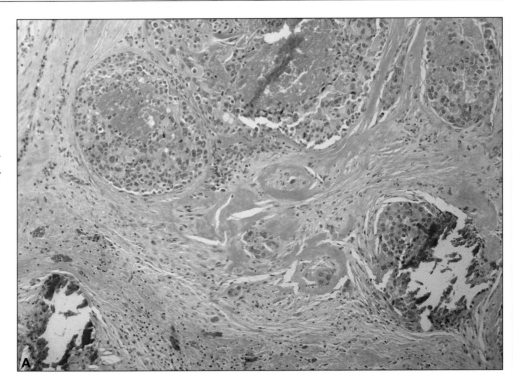

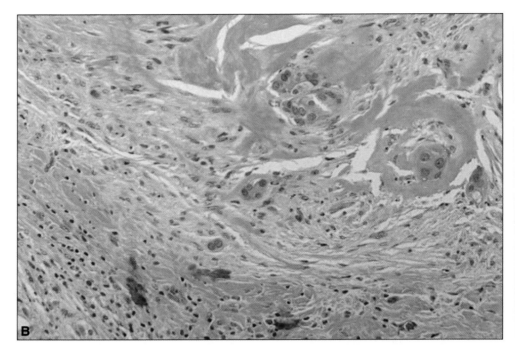

there is associated sclerosis and inflammation making the distinction between cancerization of lobules and microinvasive carcinoma difficult (Figures 9.16A,B). Microinvasive carcinoma is defined as a focus of invasive carcinoma that has a maximum dimension of less than 0.1 cm. In cases that are equivocal on hematoxylin and eosin (H&E), immunostains for myoepithelium can be useful.

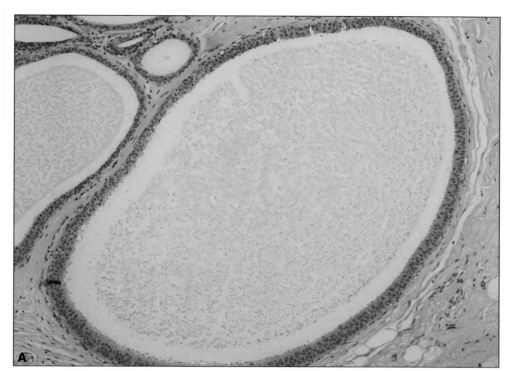

Figure 9.17. (A) Flat epithelial atypia. Dilated cystic lobules are lined by several layers of cells with low-grade cytologic atypia. Luminal secretions are evident. (B,C) Higher power view of the cells of flat epithelial atypia. The cells are relatively monotonous with round to oval nuclei with nucleolation and apical snouts. Many of the cells are maloriented to the basement membrane.

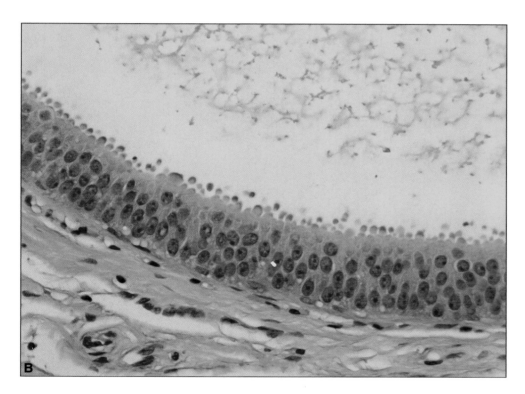

FLAT EPITHELIAL ATYPIA

FEA is a term used to encompass a particular change within the terminal ductal-lobular, which has been variably termed columnar cell change with atypia, flat

Figure 9.17. *(continued)*

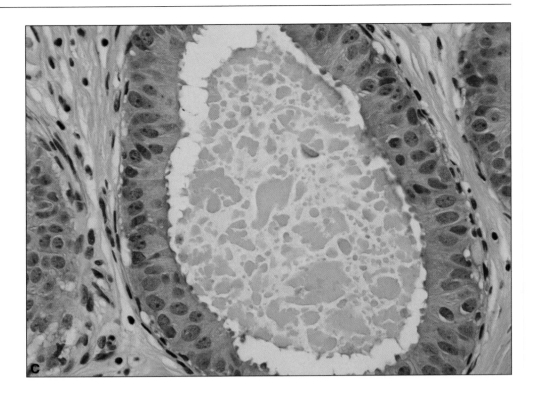

Figure 9.18. (A,B) Atypical ductal hyperplasia. Although the cells in these images resemble those of flat epithelial atypia, the micropapillary and cribriform architectural patterns take these lesions out of the spectrum of flat epithelial atypia.

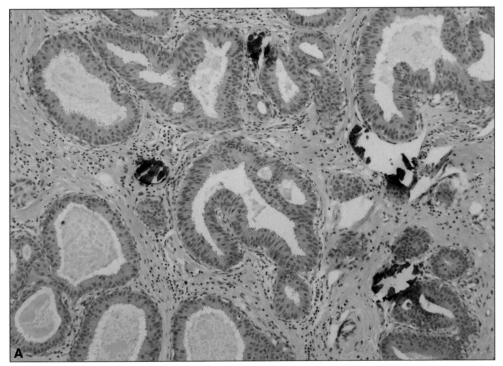

DIN-1, and clinging carcinoma to name a few. These lesions have been shown to be associated with low-grade DCIS, lobular neoplasia, and tubular carcinomas. The characteristic finding is a cluster of TDLUs, frequently associated with coarse calcifications, that are replaced by a population of monotypic, although somewhat

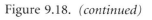

Figure 9.18. *(continued)*

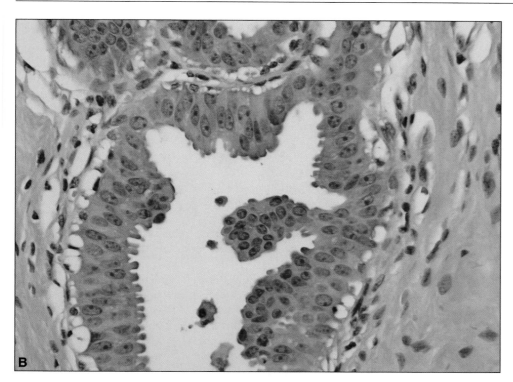

enlarged, cells with low-grade atypia (Figure 9.17A). The cells are round to oval and often have nucleoli; the cells can be several layers thick, and luminal secretions are common (Figures 9.17B,C). However, the overall low-power appearance is "flat," meaning architectural growth patterns such as micropapillae or cribriform growth are not allowed in this diagnosis (Figures 9.18A,B).

The treatment of DCIS remains complex. The current standard of care is to attempt to surgically excise DCIS with adequate margins. However, there is controversy as to what constitutes an adequate margin. Although most would agree that a margin of 1.0 cm or greater is adequate and a margin less than 0.1 cm is inadequate, the "gray" area in between has been the subject of several studies. We recommend reporting the presence of DCIS as its distance in millimeters, up to 1.0 cm, from each margin designated by the surgeon. The role of radiotherapy is also controversial, with some studies suggesting that small, non-high-grade DCIS can be treated by surgery alone with adequate margins, forgoing radiation therapy. However, the literature is conflicting and recommendations for or against radiation therapy for DCIS are best decided on a case to case basis, preferably in a multidisciplinary setting between the pathologist, surgeon, and radiation therapist. Finally, the role of estrogen receptor (ER) staining in DCIS remains controversial. Although some data has suggested only patients with ER-positive DCIS will respond to endocrine therapy, the most recent recommendation from the American Society for Clinical Oncology is that there is insufficient data to warrant routine testing of DCIS for ER.

REFERENCES

Bijker N, Peterse JL, Duchateau L, Julien JP, Fentiman IS, Duval C, et al. Risk factors for recurrence and metastasis after breast-conserving therapy for ductal carcinoma in situ: analysis of European Organization for Research and Treatment of Cancer Trial 10853. *J Clin Oncol* 2001;19(8):2263–71.

Connolly JL, Schnitt SJ, London S, Dupont W, Colditz G, Page D. Both atypical lobular hyperplasia (ALH) and atypical ductal hyperplasia (ADH) predict for bilateral breast cancer risk (Meeting abstract). *Lab Invest* 1992;66:13A.

Eusebi V, Feudale E, Foschini MP, Micheli A, Conti A, Riva C, et al. Long-term follow-up of in situ carcinoma of the breast. *Semin Diagn Pathol* 1994;11(3):223–35.

Fitzgibbons PL, Henson DE, Hutter RV. Benign breast changes and the risk for subsequent breast cancer: an update of the 1985 consensus statement. Cancer Committee of the College of American Pathologists. *Arch Pathol Lab Med* 1998;122(12):1053–5.

Goldstein NS, O'Malley BA. Cancerization of small ectatic ducts of the breast by ductal carcinoma in situ cells with apocrine snouts: a lesion associated with tubular carcinoma. *Am J Clin Pathol* 1997;107(5):561–6.

Guerra-Wallace MM, Christensen WN, White RL, Jr. A retrospective study of columnar alteration with prominent apical snouts ans secretions and the association with cancer. *Am J Surg* 2004;188(4):395–8.

Harris L, Fritsche H, Mennel R, Norton L, Ravdin P, Taube S, Somerfield MR, Hayes DF, Bast RC Jr. American Society of Clinical Oncology 2007 update of recommendations for the use of tumor markers in breast cancer. *J Clin Oncol.* 2007 Nov 20;25(33):5287–312.

Jacobs TW, Byrne C, Colditz G, Connolly JL, Schnitt SJ. Pathologic features of breast cancers in women with previous benign breast disease. *Am J Clin Pathol* 2001;115(3):362–9.

Marshall LM, Hunter DJ, Connolly JL, et al. Risk of breast cancer associated with atypical hyperplasia of lobular and ductal types. *Cancer Epidemiol Biomarkers Prev* 1997;6(5):297–301.

Page DL, Dupont WD, Rogers LW, Rados MS. Atypical hyperplastic lesions of the female breast. A long-term follow-up study. *Cancer* 1985;55(11):2698–708.

Page DL, Rogers LW. Combined histologic and cytologic criteria for the diagnosis of mammary atypical ductal hyperplasia. *Hum Pathol* 1992;23(10):1095–7.

Rosen PP. Columnar cell hyperplasia is associated with lobular carcinoma in situ and tubular carcinoma. *Am J Surg Pathol* 1999;23(12):1561.

Rosen, PP. *Rosen's Breast Pathology.* 3rd ed. Philadelphia, PA: Lippincott-Raven; 2008.

Schnitt SJ. Benign breast disease and breast cancer risk: morphology and beyond. *Am J Surg Pathol* 2003;27(6):836–41.

Schnitt SJ, Connolly JL, Tavassoli FA, et al. Interobserver reproducibility in the diagnosis of ductal proliferative breast lesions using standarized criteria [see comment]. *Am J Surg Pathol* 1992;16(12):1133–43.

Schnitt SJ, Vincent-Salomon A. Columnar cell lesions of the breast. *Adv Anat Pathol* 2003;10(3):113–24.

Tavassoli FA. Ductal intraepithelial neoplasia of the breast. *Virchows Arch* 2001;438(3):221–7.

Tavassoli FA, Hoefler H, Rosai J, Holland R, Ellis IO, Schnitt SJ, Boecker W, Heywang-Kobrunner SH, Moinfar F, Lakhani S. Intraductal Proliferative Lesions. In: Tavassoli FA, Devilee P, ed. *Pathology and Genetics: Tumours of the Breast and Female Genital Organs.* Lyon: IARC Press; 2003:63–73.

Tavassoli FA, Norris HJ. A comparison of the results of long-term follow-up for atypical intraductal hyperplasia and intraductal hyperplasia of the breast. *Cancer* 1990;65(3):518–29.

van de Vijver MJ, Peterse H. The diagnosis and management of pre-invasive breast disease: pathological diagnosis-problems with existing classification. *Breast Cancer Res* 2003;5:269.

10 INVASIVE CARCINOMA, SPECIAL TYPES

Geza Acs, MD, PhD

Introduction	137
Invasive Lobular Carcinoma	138
Tubular Carcinoma	146
Invasive Cribriform Carcinoma	151
Tubulolobular Carcinoma	154
Mucinous Carcinoma	155
Medullary Carcinoma	159
Invasive Papillary Carcinoma	162
Invasive Micropapillary Carcinoma	164
Secretory Carcinoma	170
Adenoid Cystic Carcinoma	172
Rare Histologic Patterns of Invasive Carcinoma	174
Invasive Carcinoma with Apocrine Features	174
Invasive Carcinomas with Clear Cell (Glycogen-Rich and Lipid-Rich) Features	176
Invasive Carcinoma with Signet-Ring Cell Features	177
Invasive Carcinomas with Neuroendocrine Features	178

INTRODUCTION

The special type carcinomas make up approximately 20–30 percent of all invasive breast cancers. Their frequency is generally comparable between different reported series of breast cancer, although it is higher among carcinomas detected by screening programs. The remaining invasive carcinomas are invasive ductal or no special type (NST) tumors. The diagnosis of ductal or NST carcinoma is based on the absence of histologic patterns and cytologic features, the constellation of which characterize special type carcinomas. This also means that histologic criteria for special-type carcinomas should be very well defined and strictly adhered to when making the diagnosis of any of these special types.

The main reason for the recognition of special types of invasive breast carcinoma is the improvement of prediction of likely biologic behavior beyond that provided by traditional histopathologic prognostic factors. Women diagnosed with most special type carcinomas have an excellent prognosis, often approaching that of the general population of the same age. Other special types, such as invasive micropapillary carcinoma, may suggest a particularly aggressive behavior. In addition, the various special types may be associated with unique biologic mechanisms contributing to their development and it is likely that more special types will be identified in the future, based on the combination of histologic and molecular features.

The histologic patterns, characteristic of special types of breast cancer, may be present to lesser degrees in many NST carcinomas and it is generally accepted that in order to qualify as a special type carcinoma, at least 90 percent of the tumor should be composed of the defining histologic features. Tumors with special type features present in 50–90 percent of the tumor volume can be categorized as mixed NST and special type, and the prognosis of these mixed special type tumors is often better than that of tumors with no special type features. There are two important exceptions to this rule. One exception is the carcinomas that are composed of a mixture of tubular and cribriform elements being classified according to the component making up more than 50 percent of the lesion. The other exception is carcinomas that show micropapillary features; because the presence of even a small micropapillary component within a tumor has important clinical implications (see Invasive Micropapillary Carcinoma). Obviously, tumor heterogeneity should always be kept in mind and the diagnosis of special type carcinoma should always be based on thorough sampling of the entire lesion. This also implies that a definitive diagnosis of special type carcinoma is usually not possible on core needle biopsy material. When a carcinoma on core needle biopsy shows special type features, an invasive mammary carcinoma with specific special type features should be diagnosed. It should also be emphasized here that determination and reporting of the combined histologic grade of invasive carcinomas is expected in all invasive breast carcinomas with the exception of medullary cancers.

Although some special type carcinomas, such as invasive lobular or tubular carcinoma, are relatively frequent, other special types are rarely encountered in general practice. Even though they represent less than 2 percent of all breast carcinomas, their recognition is important as they have specific clinical correlates. Other rare patterns of invasive carcinoma have also been proposed as special types of breast cancer, however at present they are not regarded as specific diagnostic entities. They are typically identified by single features, such as apocrine cytology, clear cell change or the presence of signet-ring cells that have no prognostic or clinical relevance beyond that provided by combined histologic grade and tumor stage. Nevertheless, reporting such features in otherwise NST carcinomas is relevant as it acknowledges that they have been recognized and, more importantly, that they may also be present in subsequent metastases.

INVASIVE LOBULAR CARCINOMA

Invasive lobular carcinoma (ILC) is the second most common type of invasive mammary carcinoma. Its frequency varies widely in reported series from less than 1 percent up to 15 percent. This wide variation is most likely due to differences in diagnostic criteria used. Some recent reports suggested that the frequency of ILC is increasing; however, these studies are based on registry data and given the inconsistency of diagnostic criteria applied, more studies are needed to confirm these observations. In addition, the recognition of variants of ILC may have also contributed to the reported increased frequency in recent reports. Other studies suggested that postmenopausal patients receiving combined hormone therapy may have an increased risk of ILC; however, other studies indicate that the increased risk is more associated with low grade rather than specific histologic type of tumors.

Clinical Features

The average age at presentation with ILC is 60–64 years. As with NST carcinoma, ILC may present as a palpable mass or mammographic abnormality, although it is less likely to be associated with mammographic microcalcifications. Although the majority of ILCs exhibit a distinct tumor mass, which is easily detected both radiologically and macroscopically, some of these tumors grow diffusely, representing a vague area of thickening or palpable induration of the breast tissue without distinct limits. The latter cases may be difficult to detect clinically or mammographically, and the size of the tumor and extent of the disease are frequently underestimated. Multifocality, multicentricity, and bilaterality are frequently occurring characteristics of ILC. Although the frequency of multicentric ILC varies between 9 and 31 percent in various reports, Tot found that multifocal tumors were more often lobular (25 percent) compared to unifocal tumors (4 percent), in a detailed analysis of the distribution of invasive breast carcinoma using large-format histologic sections. He reported that approximately 12 percent of his ILC cases were multifocal, which is a lower proportion in comparison to some other studies, and suggested that some diffuse tumors (see Treatment and Prognosis) were classified as multifocal in some studies that did not use large-format histologic sections.

Macroscopic and Microscopic Features

The gross appearance of ILC may be similar to NST carcinomas as it may form a spiculated, gray, firm mass. In other cases of low cellularity tumors with a diffuse spread in the breast tissue, gross examination may reveal little or no discernable abnormality. The average size at presentation is 2.4 cm, however in tumors characterized by diffuse spread, the size of the lesion can be difficult to determine.

Similar to other special types, more than 90 percent of the carcinoma should have a lobular morphology to be classified as ILC. The characteristic cells of ILC are small, with scant cytoplasm and round or ovoid, bland nuclei that are often eccentrically placed (Figure 10.1). Intracytoplasmic lumina, which can be highlighted with periodic acid Schiff (PAS) or mucicarmine stains, are relatively frequently found in cells of ILC and occasionally may be prominent (Figure 10.2). In addition to classic ILC, several variants or subtypes have been identified based on the differences in histological growth pattern and cytologic atypia. The most common pattern is the classic variant (approximately 40 percent), which is characterized by a single-cell infiltrating pattern (Figure 10.3). The neoplastic cells form single files and often encircle existing normal ducts in a targetoid fashion. The second most common variant is the solid type, representing approximately 10 percent of ILC. In this variant the characteristic cells infiltrate the breast tissue in large solid sheets or irregularly shaped nests with little intervening stroma

Figure 10.1. Invasive lobular carcinoma, classic type. The characteristic tumor cells are small, with scant cytoplasm and round, bland nuclei. The neoplastic cells infiltrate in single files.

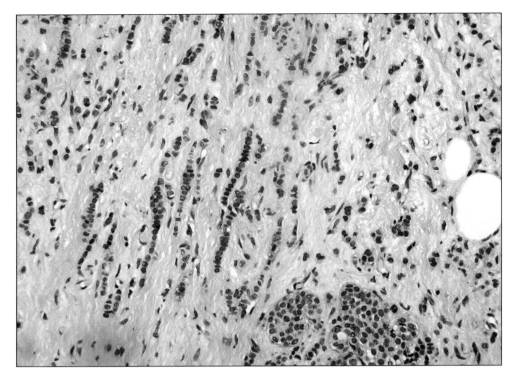

Figure 10.2. Intracytoplasmic lumina can sometimes be prominent in cells of invasive lobular carcinoma.

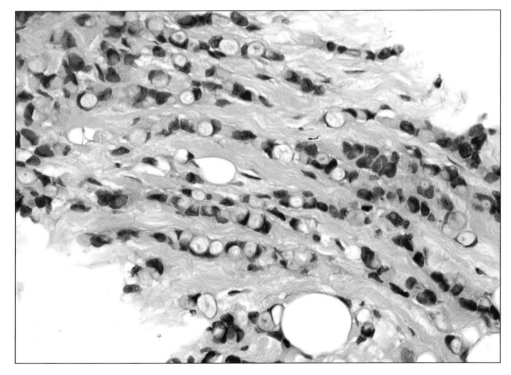

(Figure 10.4). In the alveolar variant, which accounts for only 4–5 percent of ILC, the tumor cells grow in well-defined, round aggregates composed of twenty cells or more (Figure 10.5). ILC can be classified into one of the specific subtypes if at least 80 percent of the tumor shows a single pattern. Otherwise, cases can be classified as

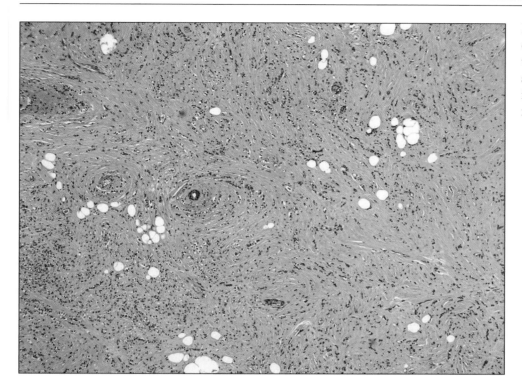

Figure 10.3. Invasive lobular carcinoma, classic type. The tumor is sparsely cellular with small, bland neoplastic cells infiltrating is a single file manner.

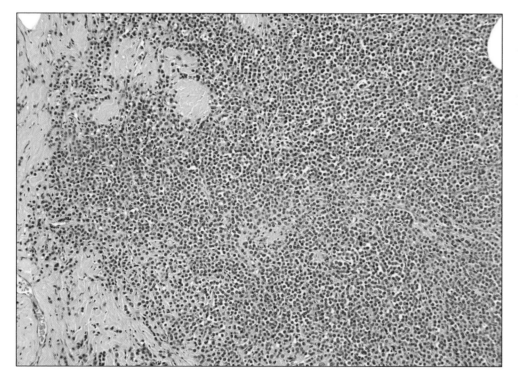

Figure 10.4. Invasive lobular carcinoma, solid type. In this variant the characteristic dyscohesive neoplastic cells infiltrate the breast tissue in large solid sheets or irregularly shaped nests.

ILC with mixed pattern, which group accounts for about 40 percent. Most ILCs are of low or intermediate combined histologic grade, scoring 3 for lack of tubule formation, 1 or 2 for nuclear pleomorphism and 1 for typically low mitotic rate. Recently, the term "pleomorphic invasive lobular carcinoma" (PILC) has been

Figure 10.5. Invasive lobular carcinoma, alveolar type. The tumor cells show the characteristic features of lobular carcinoma, but grow in well-defined, round aggregates composed of twenty cells or more.

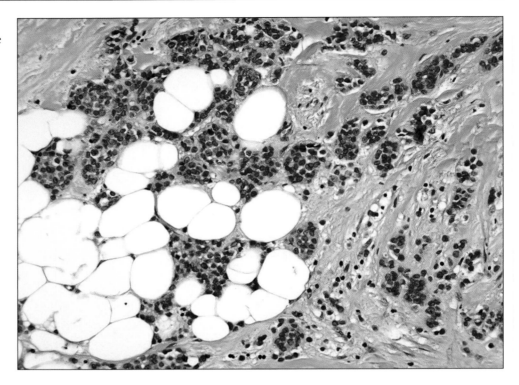

introduced to describe invasive carcinomas that show any of the characteristic growth patterns of lobular carcinoma described earlier, but have grade III, highly atypical nuclei, and sometimes increased mitotic activity (Figure 10.6). A proportion of PILC also feature apocrine differentiation as evidenced by abundant, eosinophilic cytoplasm and prominent nucleoli (Figure 10.7). The term pleomorphic is descriptive, and for clinical purposes the combined histologic grade of the tumor should be documented, differing from other ILC by high nuclear grade. Lobular carcinoma in situ (LCIS) is associated in 66 percent of cases (up to 90 percent in the case of the classic type), whereas ductal carcinoma in situ (DCIS) (usually low grade) is seen in about 14 percent.

In general, ILC is more likely to be hormone receptor–positive compared to NST carcinoma; estrogen receptor (ER) expression is present in 92 percent and progesterone (PR) expression in 60–70 percent of the cases, respectively. On the other hand, ILCs, with the exception of PILC, are generally HER2/neu negative. ILCs, including PILCs, show a characteristic loss or marked reduction of E-cadherin membrane expression in the vast majority of cases. The E-cadherin gene (CDH1) located on 16q22 has been shown to be mutated or lost in ILC. In a proportion of cases the loss of E-cadherin expression is attributed to promoter methylation, which is potentially reversible. ILC in general shows a lower number of chromosomal changes compared to NST tumors (6.4 vs. 10.1). Characteristic chromosomal alterations in ILC include the loss of 16q (63 percent) and gain of 1q (79 percent).

Differential Diagnosis

There is little difficulty in establishing the diagnosis in ILC cases showing classic cytologic features and growth pattern. However, focal single-cell infiltrating

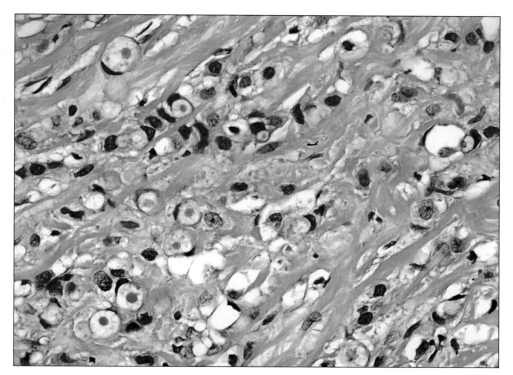

Figure 10.6. Pleomorphic invasive lobular carcinoma. The tumor shows an infiltrative pattern characteristic of lobular carcinoma, but the constituent cells exhibit marked pleomoprhism. Signet-ring cell features are not uncommonly found in association with higher nuclear grades in lobular cancers.

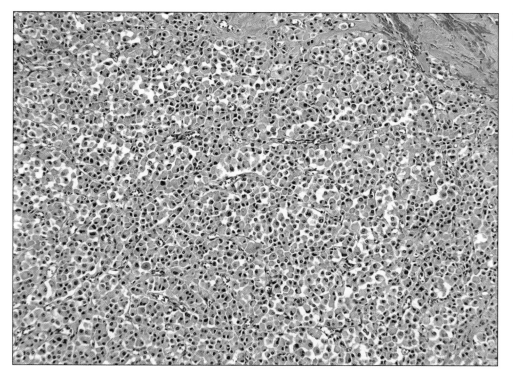

Figure 10.7. Pleomorphic invasive lobular carcinoma with apocrine features. The carcinoma shows a dyscohesive, solid growth pattern and is composed of large tumor cells with atypical nuclei and abundant eosinophilic cytoplasm.

pattern or targetoid growth may frequently be found in otherwise NST carcinoma. These focal areas in an otherwise NST carcinoma usually retain E-cadherin positivity and their presence does not warrant a diagnosis of a mixed type tumor. We prefer to classify the tumors that exhibit a true biphasic pattern composed of

Figure 10.8. (A) Invasive carcinoma, mixed ductal NST and lobular type. The NST component of the carcinoma is composed of cohesive nests and glands, whereas the distinct lobular component shows dyscohesive cells growing in a single-file infiltrative pattern.
(B) E-cadherin immunostaining shows strong membrane reactivity in the NST carcinoma component and complete lack of staining in the lobular component.

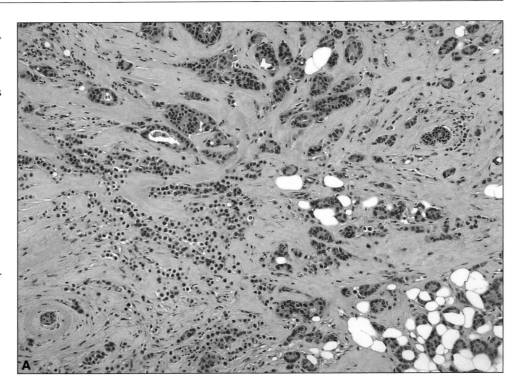

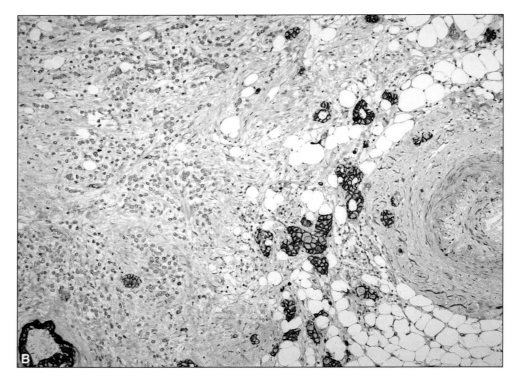

characteristic lobular and other elements as mixed lobular and NST (or other special type), which is also usually reflected in differential E-cadherin staining patterns (Figures 10.8A,B). The distinction between PILC and NST carcinoma may be particularly difficult, and if focal gland formation, cohesive trabecular growth

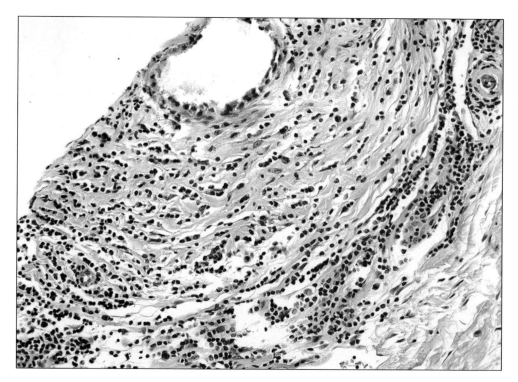

Figure 10.9. Sclerosis and chronic inflammation around a small duct. The lymphocytes form single files and show targetoid patterns around the benign duct mimicking invasive lobular carcinoma.

pattern, and diffuse E-cadherin positivity are present, the diagnosis of PILC should be reconsidered.

Although E-cadherin staining is a useful tool in the differential diagnosis of ILC, "aberrant" diffuse or focal membrane expression of E-cadherin may be present in a significant number of ILC cases and a diagnosis of ductal (NST) carcinoma should not be based solely on the presence of E-cadherin immunopositivity in a tumor otherwise exhibiting lobular morphology. On the other hand, in our experience complete loss of E-cadherin staining is exceedingly rare in NST cancers.

An important differential diagnosis is presented by paucicellular ILC that does not form a mass lesion and is not recognized grossly or microscopically. Focal grouping of small cells in the breast stroma should always raise the possibility of ILC and the presence of tumor cells can be confirmed using immunohistochemical stains for cytokeratins or epithelial membrane antigen (EMA).

The solid variant of ILC may raise the differential diagnosis of lymphoma or plasmacytoma. Clinical history and the use of appropriate immunostains for lymphoid and epithelial markers may help the pathologist render the correct diagnosis. Rarely, sclerosis and chronic inflammation around ductal structures may mimic ILC (Figure 10.9), and the use of immunohistochemical stains may be required in these settings.

Treatment and Prognosis

At the time of presentation, 32–43 percent of patients with ILC have axillary lymph node metastases, and about 8 percent have distant metastases. Compared to NST carcinomas, ILC is associated with particular patterns of distant metastases, showing frequent involvement of peritoneal surfaces, the female genital tract, and the gastrointestinal tract.

There is controversy regarding the prognosis of ILC compared to NST carcinomas, which can at least partly be attributed to inconsistent use of diagnostic criteria. In general, improved survival was found for low-grade classic ILC cases, the prognosis of which appear to be favorable (70–80 percent five-year survival) compared to NST tumors. Without separation of low grade from other ILC cases, recent series showed no significant difference between overall survival, local or distant recurrence rates compared to nonlobular type carcinomas.

A recent meta-analysis with long follow-up suggested that although ILCs are associated with an early advantage in disease-free and overall survival compared to NST cases (at 6 years), a late advantage was found for the NST cohort after 10 years of follow-up consistent with late recurrences in the ILC group. This is most likely due to the usually extremely slow growth of ILC. The importance of the prognostic significance of grade is emphasized by studies of PILC that are associated with aggressive behavior. Besides combined histologic grade, histologic subtype and growth pattern also appear to have prognostic significance. The solid variant of ILC appears to have a poor prognosis showing association with 82 percent locoregional and 54 percent distant recurrence rates, and 47 percent twelve-year survival.

Although ILC is frequently multifocal (Figure 10.10A) and bilateral, this alone does not appear to have a bearing on the outcome. In contrast, some observations suggest that the diffuse growth pattern of ILCs may have clinical and prognostic relevance. The diffuse growth pattern, defined as small tumors simultaneously developing in a large number of neighboring terminal duct-lobular units and/or exhibiting a nonlobulocentric growth resulting in the tumor having an appearance resembling that of a spider's web in large histological sections (Figure 10.10B), is present in approximately one-third of ILC cases. In addition to being associated with increased frequency of positive margins, tumors exhibiting a diffuse growth pattern had a significantly higher rate of cancer-related death than the other groups (25 vs. 6–8 percent). In addition to larger tumor size, delay in detection and clinical and morphological understaging of the disease in these cases may explain the adverse prognosis. The introduction of the diagnostic category of ILC exhibiting a diffuse growth pattern was suggested to highlight the unique features and clinical implications of these tumors.

TUBULAR CARCINOMA

Tubular carcinoma constitutes 1–7 percent of invasive breast carcinomas, depending on the strictness of criteria used to diagnose this special type. However, among breast cancers detected in screening programs, much higher frequencies, up to 19 percent of cases, were reported.

Clinical Features

Patients with tubular carcinoma present at an average age of 58–65 years. Mammographically it appears as an irregular, spiculated mass lesion. Approximately, 20 percent of cases were reported to be multifocal.

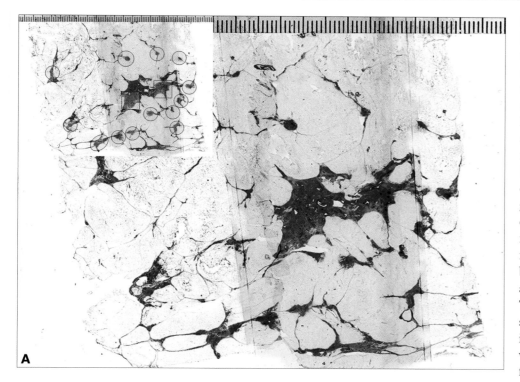

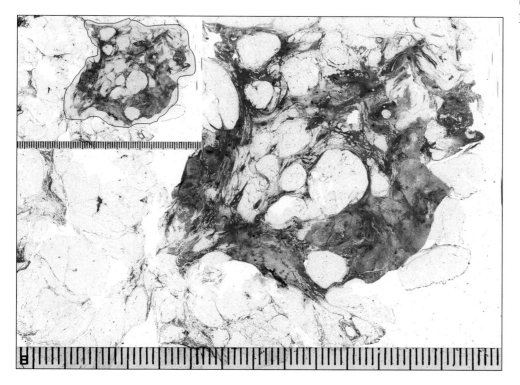

Figure 10.10. (A) Multifocal invasive lobular carcinoma shows distinct tumor nodules separate from each other, which can be best demonstrated by large format histologic section. The shaded areas in the inset mark the multiple distinct tumor foci. (B) Invasive lobular carcinoma with diffuse growth pattern. The tumor exhibits a diffuse, nonlobulocentric growth with no discernable tumor masses but rather resembles the appearance of a spider's web. This growth pattern may be seen in up to one-third of invasive lobular carcinoma when examined by large format histologic sections. (Courtesy of Dr. Tibor Tot, Falun, Sweden).

Macroscopic and Microscopic Features

Macroscopically there are no specific features that differentiate tubular carcinoma from NST tumors. The tumors are generally small, between 0.2 to 2 cm, with the

Figure 10.11. Tubular carcinoma. The tumor is composed entirely of open, angulated tubules lined by a single layer of epithelial cells.

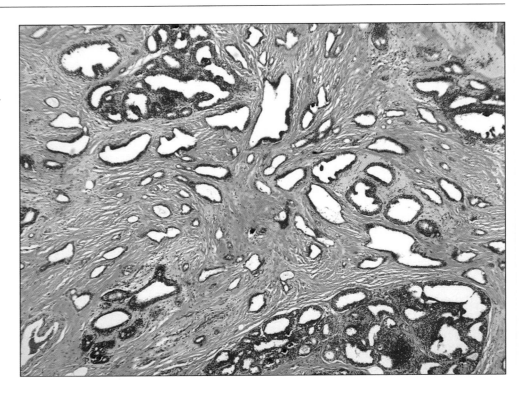

majority measuring 1 cm or less. Larger tumors are often mixed with NST elements. The tumors are generally hard, fixed to the surrounding tissue, and show a stellate, gray mass lesion on slicing.

Microscopically, tubular carcinoma is characterized by the presence of well-formed, angulated or tear-drop-shaped tubules with open lumina (Figure 10.11). The tubules are distributed randomly and are associated with a desmoplastic stroma. The tubules frequently infiltrate between the benign structures and the adipose tissue. The center of the lesion may show hyalinized fibrosis containing scanty tubules. The tubules are characteristically lined by a single layer of low-grade, bland epithelial cells with round nuclei, usually without nucleoli (Figure 10.12). Nuclear atypia is mild to moderate and mitotic activity is low or unapparent. By definition, tubular carcinoma is of low combined histologic grade with a combined score of 3 or 4. Frequently, but not uniformly, the lining epithelial cells have apical apocrine snouts and the lumina may contain secretions (Figure 10.13). The diagnosis of pure tubular carcinoma requires the presence of the characteristic features in more than 90 percent of the tumor and the lack of high-grade cytologic atypia. Tumors showing 50–90 percent tubular features are classified as mixed tubular and NST carcinoma. The exceptions to this rule are carcinomas composed of tubular and cribriform elements, by which tumors can be typed as pure tubular if more than 50 percent of the lesion is composed of tubular pattern and the rest of the tumor has the morphology of invasive cribriform carcinoma (see Invasive Cribriform Carcinoma) with no high-grade elements.

The majority of cases have associated DCIS, usually low grade with cribriform or micropapillary pattern. In addition, a frequent association with lobular neoplasia and columnar cell change/hyperplasia with or without atypia has been reported in several studies. These associations may suggest similar pathways for

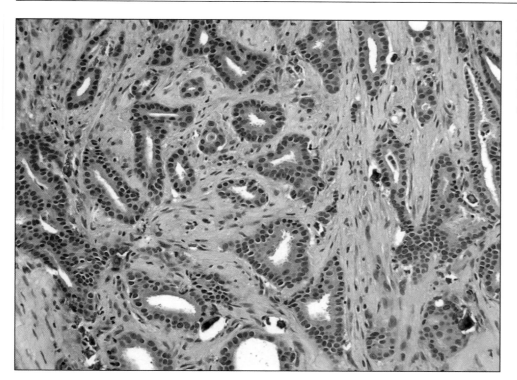

Figure 10.12. Tubular carcinoma. The tubules are lined by a single layer of bland epithelial cells with round nuclei and are associated with a desmoplastic stroma.

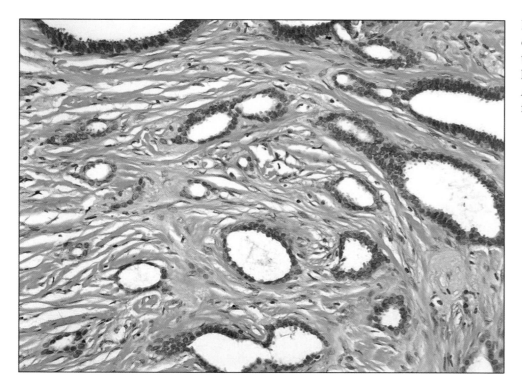

Figure 10.13. Tubular carcinoma. The angulated tubules are lined by a single layer of bland epithelial cells. Apical apocrine snouts are frequently present.

tumor development for tubular and lobular carcinomas. The frequent presence of chromosomal changes, such as the loss of 16q (34 percent) and gain of 1q (50 percent), similar to those characteristic of ILC, may also support this hypothesis. Tubular carcinomas are ER- and PR-positive in more than 90 and 75 percent

Figure 10.14. Tubular carcinoma. The infiltration of the open tubules between normal structures and into adipose tissue is a helpful diagnostic feature.

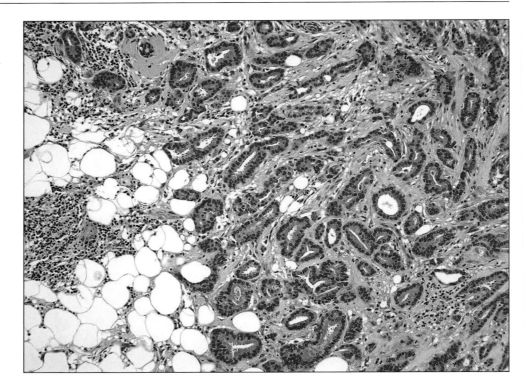

of the cases, respectively, and HER2/neu-negative in more than 95 percent of the cases.

Differential Diagnosis

The main differential diagnosis includes complex sclerosing lesions (CSL) and sclerosing adenosis. CSL have a stellate configuration with radial arrangement of tubular elements, usually trapped in the central elastotic scar. However, the tubules show the presence of myoepithelial cells and there is a lack of a desmoplastic response. Infiltration of "naked" tubules into surrounding adipose tissue is a useful diagnostic feature of tubular carcinoma (Figure 10.14). In contrast to the irregular infiltration of open, angulated tubules seen in tubular carcinoma, sclerosing adenosis maintains a lobulocentric configuration at low-power examination and the glandular spaces tend to be compressed with maintenance of a double-cell layer. When necessary, the absence of myoepithelial cells in tubular carcinoma can be confirmed with appropriate markers such as smooth muscle myosin heavy chain, p63, or calponin.

Microglandular adenosis (MGA) may also superficially mimic tubular carcinoma. In MGA, small round glands with an apparent single layer of epithelial lining infiltrate the stroma and adipose tissue in an irregular, nonlobulocentric fashion. The usually angulated shape of the tubules in tubular carcinoma is in contrast with the regular, round glands in MGA. The lack of an associated desmoplastic stromal response in MGA also helps in establishing the correct diagnosis.

Treatment and Prognosis

Although axillary lymph node metastases were reported in 12–30 percent of tubular carcinoma, distant metastases and tumor related death are extremely rare. Nodal metastases, when present, usually involve only a small number of nodes (1–3). The rate of local recurrence was reported to be 1–10 percent in patients with tubular carcinoma, which compares favorably to those seen in low grade NST cancers. The development of local recurrence in these cases is somewhat confusing, since tubular carcinomas may be multifocal in a significant number of cases and it is not clear whether the "recurrence" simply represents multifocal disease. Nevertheless, local recurrence does not appear to significantly worsen the excellent prognosis associated with the diagnosis of pure tubular carcinoma; the five-year and overall survival rates are 94 and 88 percent, respectively, which compare favorably with an age-matched control population. It is generally accepted that pure tubular carcinomas less than 1 cm in size can be treated by excision alone.

INVASIVE CRIBRIFORM CARCINOMA

Invasive cribriform carcinoma is closely related to tubular carcinoma both histologically and biologically, although less frequently recognized by pathologists as a special type in practice. Invasive cribriform carcinoma is uncommon, representing 0.8–3.5 percent of breast cancers. As in the case of other special type carcinomas, its incidence is higher in the mammographically screened population.

Clinical Features

The clinical and mammographic presentation of invasive cribriform carcinoma does not differ significantly from that of NST carcinomas. These tumors may present at a larger size compared to tubular carcinoma, with an average diameter of 3 cm. The average age at presentation is 53–58 years. Radiographically, they appear as spiculated masses with frequent associated microcalcifications.

Macroscopic and Microscopic Features

Invasive cribriform carcinomas have no specific gross features to distinguish them from usual breast carcinomas.

This type of carcinoma infiltrates the stroma as islands of cells forming punched-out spaces reminiscent of cribriform-type DCIS (Figure 10.15). The infiltrating islands are of irregular shape and variable size and usually a desmoplastic stromal reaction is present. The constituent cells are small and uniform with grade I or grade II nuclei, and by and large resemble the cells of tubular carcinoma (Figure 10.16). Apical apocrine snouts may be present. The cribriform spaces may be replaced focally by solid nests of tumor cells, but the cytologic features of the tumor cells remain similar. In some tumors, an apparent second cell population may be present composed of cells with more abundant, pale cytoplasm, but similar nuclear features (Figure 10.17). These cells are present dispersed singly or in small clusters and may resemble cells of lobular neoplasia, although there is no evidence for their lobular differentiation. Associated DCIS, usually low grade, cribriform type, is present in 80 percent of the cases. These tumors are ER-positive in virtually

Figure 10.15. Invasive cribriform carcinoma. Islands of tumor cells forming punched-out spaces reminiscent of cribriform-type ductal carcinoma in situ infiltrate the stroma. Note the presence of a desmoplastic stromal reaction.

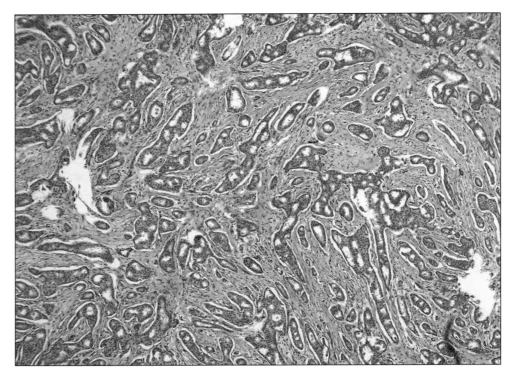

Figure 10.16. Invasive cribriform carcinoma. The constituent cells are small and uniform with grade 1 or 2 nuclei. Apical apocrine snouts may be present.

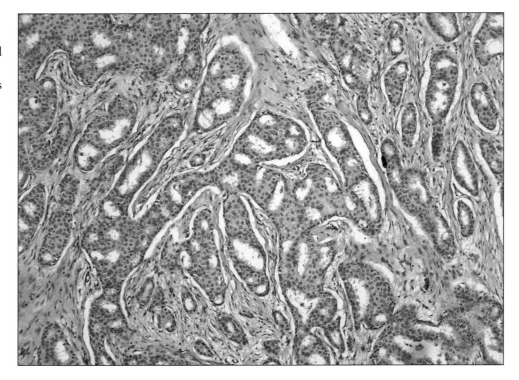

100 percent of cases, PR positivity is about 70 percent and they do not overexpress HER2/neu.

The diagnosis of invasive cribriform carcinoma requires the presence of the characteristic features in more than 90 percent of the tumor and lack of high-grade

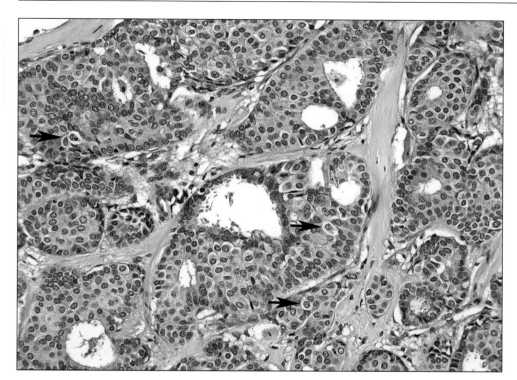

Figure 10.17. Invasive cribriform carcinoma. In some cases an apparent second cell population may be present composed of cells with more abundant, pale cytoplasm, but similar nuclear features. These pale cells can be dispersed (arrows) or sometimes form small nests.

cytologic atypia. Tumors showing 50–90 percent cribriform features are classified as mixed types. As in the case of tubular carcinoma, tumors composed of tubular and cribriform elements can be classified as cribriform if more than 50 percent of the lesion displays this pattern.

Differential Diagnosis

The main differential diagnosis is cribriform ductal carcinoma in situ, whose distinction may be difficult if sclerosis, scarring, and distortion are present. Besides the irregular shape and varying size of the nests, and the presence of a desmoplastic stromal reaction in invasive cribriform carcinoma, infiltration of tumor-cell nests within adipose tissue or beyond the confines of lobular units may signify an invasive process. In addition, in invasive cribriform carcinoma the tumor-cell islands lack a myoepithelial-cell layer.

Adenoid cystic carcinoma (ACC) may sometimes present a differential diagnostic challenge. ACC is characterized by a dual cell population forming two types of crisp spaces (see Adenoid Cystic Carcinoma). Alcian blue/periodic acid Schiff (AB/PAS) stain may help highlight the two types of spaces, and immunohistochemical stains for myoepithelial and epithelial markers highlight the two-cell population in ACC. The uniform lack of hormone receptor expression in ACC is in contrast with the almost 100 percent ER positivity of invasive cribriform carcinoma and may also be useful in this distinction. Rare invasive neuroendocrine carcinomas metastatic to or primary in the breast can be excluded by appropriate immunohistochemical stains for neuroendocrine markers.

Treatment and Prognosis

Axillary lymph node metastases are seen in 14–37 percent of cases. Metastatic carcinomas tend to involve low numbers (1–3) of nodes and retain the histological features of the primary tumor. Distant metastases are extremely rare. With a median follow-up of 14.5 years, Page and coworkers saw no tumor-related deaths in pure invasive cribriform carcinomas. This excellent prognosis, even when nodal metastasis is present, was also confirmed in subsequent studies.

TUBULOLOBULAR CARCINOMA

Tubulolobular carcinoma was first described by Fisher and colleagues in 1977 as a tubular variant of lobular carcinoma. Some authors place this type of carcinoma within the category of a variant of ILC. Although this approach may be appropriate, tubulolobular carcinomas show unique characteristics that distinguish them from other variants of lobular carcinoma and their definitive classification remains elusive, justifying their discussion here as a separate special type of breast cancer.

Clinical Features

Tubulolobular carcinomas are rare, accounting for less than 2 percent of invasive breast cancers. Patients present at an average age of 59–60 years (range 43–79 years). The tumors tend to be small on presentation and are firm with slightly irregular borders. Multifocality has been reported in 19–29 percent of the cases.

Macroscopic and Microscopic Features

There are no specific gross features that distinguish this special type from other mammary carcinomas. The tumors measure from 0.5 to 2.5 cm (median 1.4 cm) and are usually described as firm, indurated gray/tan masses.

Microscopically the tumor is composed of intermixed small, round tubular structures and single-cell strands of tumor cells infiltrating in a fashion reminiscent of ILC, often with targetoid arrangements around benign structures (Figures 10.18). The tubules are round and usually much smaller than the angulated tubules seen in tubular carcinoma, but are also lined by a single layer of epithelial cells. The neoplastic cells are small with scant cytoplasm and usually round, bland, low-grade nuclei. These tumors show low mitotic activity and are of low combined histologic grade, usually with a combined score of 4 or 5. The stroma is densely collagenous with prominent elastosis. An in-situ element, usually low-grade DCIS with a cribriform or micropapillary pattern, is often present; however, associated lobular neoplasia can also be found. Similar to other special type cancers, more than 90 percent of the tumor should show the characteristic pattern to be classified as tubulolobular carcinoma.

These tumors are hormone receptor–positive in the vast majority of cases and do not show HER2 overexpression. In contrast to other variants of lobular carcinoma, all reported cases of tubulolobular carcinomas showed strong membrane expression of E-cadherin and p120 catenin.

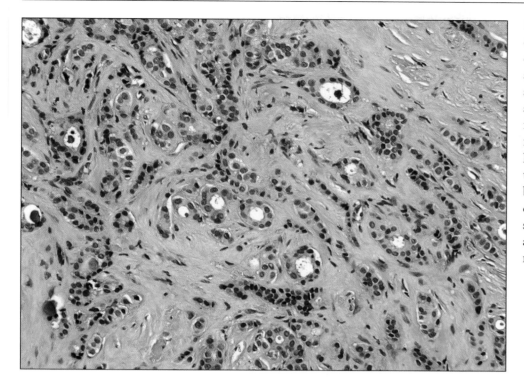

Figure 10.18. Tubulolobular carcinoma. The tumor is composed of intermixed small, round tubular structures and single-cell strands of tumor cells infiltrating in a fashion reminiscent of invasive lobular carcinoma. The tubules are round and lined by a single layer of epithelial cells. The neoplastic cells are small with scant cytoplasm and round, bland, low-grade nuclei.

Differential Diagnosis

Tubulolobular carcinomas must be distinguished from tubular carcinomas and carcinomas composed of distinct tubular and lobular carcinoma components (mixed tubular and lobular carcinomas). In tubulolobular carcinoma, the tubules are round and of small size in contrast with the larger, angulated open tubules of tubular carcinoma. The intimate admixture of the small round tubules and single-cell cords, both of which show a lobular pattern infiltration, distinguishes tubulo-lobular carcinomas from mixed tubular and lobular carcinomas, which usually show distinct separate components of tubular and lobular carcinoma (Figure 10.19A,B). The lobular component in the latter cases is typically E-cadherin-negative.

Treatment and Prognosis

Tubulolobular carcinomas are associated with regional lymph node and distant metastases in about 13–17 and 13 percent of the cases, respectively. Although a small number of cases have been reported, the prognosis for this special type appears to be between pure tubular and classic ILC.

MUCINOUS CARCINOMA

Invasive mucinous carcinomas are relatively uncommon in their pure form, accounting for 1–6 percent of invasive carcinomas. In contrast to other good prognosis special type cancers, mucinous carcinomas are not found with increased frequency in series with mammographic screening.

155

Figure 10.19. (A) Mixed tubular and lobular carcinoma. The tumor shows areas of tubular carcinoma with characteristic angulated tubules, whereas other areas are composed of classic invasive lobular carcinoma. In contrast to tubulolobular carcinoma that shows an intimate admixture of small round tubules and single file infiltration, the tubular and lobular elements appear to be separate in these cases. (B) E-cadherin immunostains highlight the separate tubular and lobular elements. Tubulolobular carcinomas are usually diffusely E-cadherin-positive.

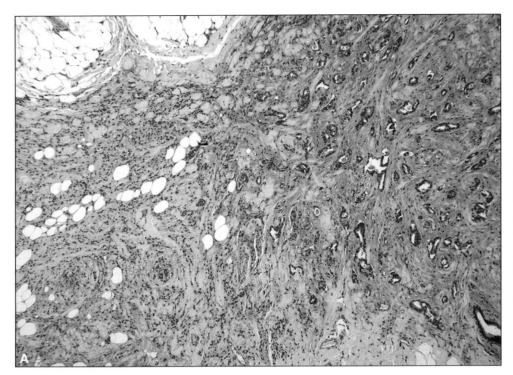

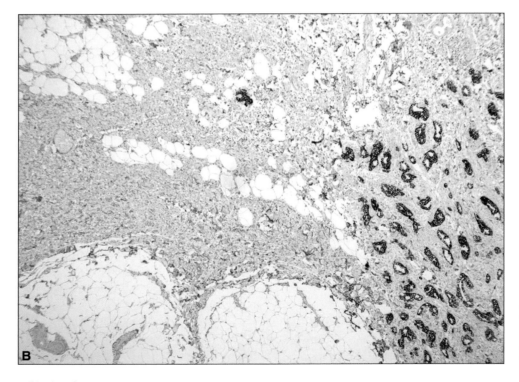

Clinical Features

Patients with mucinous carcinoma tend to be postmenopausal with a mean age of 59–71 years, and usually present with a palpable mass. Mammographically, these tumors are usually seen as well-circumscribed, often benign-appearing mass lesions.

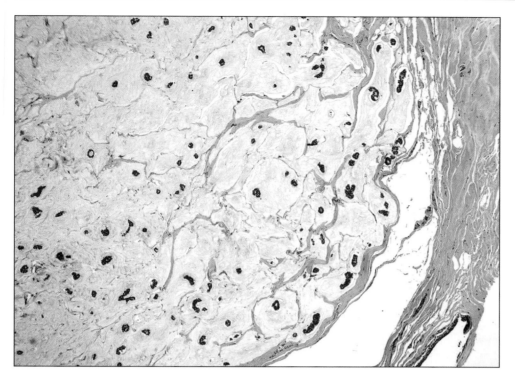

Figure 10.20. Mucinous carcinoma. The tumor is characterized by the presence of abundant extracellular pools of mucin in which nests, glands, and trabeculae of tumor cells appear to be floating. Mucinous carcinomas are usually sharply circumscribed.

Macroscopic and Microscopic Features

Mucinous carcinomas measure 1–4 cm, but much larger examples have also been reported. Macroscopically they form well-circumscribed, smooth, rounded masses that have a glistening, gelatinous cut surface.

Microscopically these tumors are characterized by the presence of abundant extracellular pools of mucin, which usually comprise more than 50 percent of the tumor volume (Figure 10.20). The tumors are usually sharply circumscribed, although focal infiltration of the surrounding stroma may be seen. The tumor cells, arranged in small trabeculae, nests, or glands with central lumens, appear to float in the mucin (Figure 10.21). Cellularity is variable. The tumor cells have moderate amounts of eosinophilic, granular cytoplasm and may contain intracellular mucin. A mucin-producing DCIS may also be present. Nuclear atypia is generally mild. Indeed, some authorities regard a low nuclear grade as a prerequisite for the diagnosis of pure mucinous carcinoma and diagnose similar tumors with higher grade nuclei as NST carcinomas with mucinous features (Figure 10.22).

Mucinous carcinomas are ER- and PR-positive in 73–95 and 79–84 percent of cases, respectively, and tend to be negative for HER2/neu overexpression. Argyrophilic granules and immunohistochemical positivity for neuroendocrine markers can be identified, but does not appear to have any clinical or prognostic significance. Recently, nuclear expression of WT1 was also reported in mucinous carcinomas.

Differential Diagnosis

Mucinous carcinomas should be distinguished from mucocele-like lesions. These lesions usually show acellular pools of mucin with dissection of collagen bundles in

Figure 10.21. Mucinous carcinoma. The tumor cells arranged in small trabeculae, nests, or glands with central lumens appearing to float in the mucin. The tumor cells have moderate amounts of eosinophilic cytoplasm and may contain intracellular mucin. Nuclear atypia is generally mild.

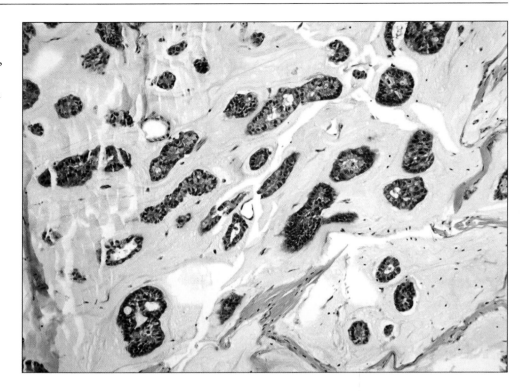

Figure 10.22. Tumors with extracellular mucin but high-grade nuclear features are diagnosed as NST carcinomas with mucinous features, rather than pure mucinous carcinomas.

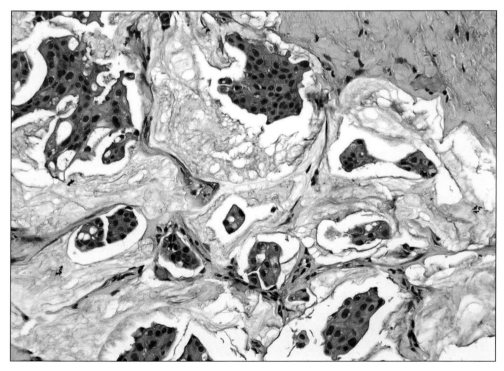

the connective tissue, which contrasts with the usually well-circumscribed borders of mucinous carcinoma. Sometimes mucocele-like lesions show cysts lined by proliferating atypical cells and occasional mucin-producing in situ carcinomas may be associated with rupture and extracellular mucin. Differentiation in these rare cases may be difficult and one should search for areas of clearly diagnosable invasive carcinoma.

Invasive NST carcinomas can present with focal areas of extracellular mucin pools. The characteristic mucinous features should be present in more than 90 percent of the tumor to be classified as a mucinous carcinoma; otherwise a diagnosis of NST carcinoma with focal mucinous features should be rendered.

Invasive micropapillary carcinomas may also have extracellular mucin and are sometimes confused with mucinous carcinomas. The mucin pools in these latter cases are usually less abundant, the tumors are more cellular and the tumor-cell nests retain their characteristic micropapillary morphology (see Invasive Micropapillary Carcinoma). This feature can also be highlighted by immunohistochemical stains for EMA.

Treatment and Prognosis

Regional lymph node metastasis is seen in only 14 percent of cases. When the diagnosis is restricted to low-grade lesions, mucinous carcinomas are associated with an excellent prognosis. The five-year disease-free and disease-specific survival rates are 81–90 and 95.3 percent, respectively. However, this survival rate significantly drops on long-term follow-up.

MEDULLARY CARCINOMA

Medullary carcinoma was established as a special type carcinoma because of its relatively favorable prognosis despite its high-grade histologic features. In recent years, it has gained additional interest due to its association with BRCA1-related breast cancers. Medullary carcinoma is the only special type cancer that is exempt from the requirement of combined histologic grading, because its histologic and cytologic features along with high proliferative activity are in contrast with its favorable prognostic implications.

Clinical Features

Medullary carcinoma accounts for 1–10 percent of all invasive breast carcinomas in different series. The wide variation in frequency most likely reflects variation in the strictness of criteria used for the diagnosis. Medullary carcinomas present over a wide age range, however, they tend to present at a younger age than carcinomas overall with about half of the patients being less than 50 years of age. These tumors may appear benign both clinically and mammographically because of their smooth borders and sharp demarcation from the stroma. The typical mammographic appearance is a round, sharply circumscribed mass without calcifications.

Macroscopic and Microscopic Features

Medullary carcinomas usually measure between 1 and 4 cm in greatest diameter and have a characteristic gross appearance. These tumors are well circumscribed with a

Figure 10.23. Medullary carcinoma. The tumor is composed of interconnecting sheets of high-grade tumor cells with abundant cytoplasm and indistinct cell borders (syncytial growth pattern). The stroma between the sheets of tumor cells contains a diffuse, moderate to marked lymphoplasmacytic infiltrate.

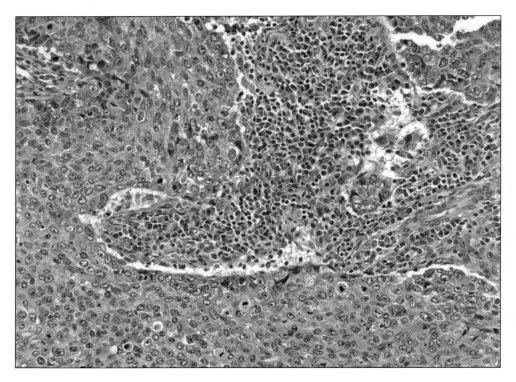

soft, gray/white cut surface. Foci of hemorrhage, necrosis, or central cystification may be present.

Although the histologic features of medullary carcinoma have been debated in the literature, the best description still comes from Ridolfi's original publication of their series. The essential histologic features include a syncytial growth pattern involving more than 75 percent of the tumor mass. This characteristic growth pattern includes interconnecting sheets of tumor cells with abundant cytoplasm and indistinct cell borders (Figure 10.23). No gland formation or trabecular growth is present. The tumor cells are large with pleomorphic nuclei, clumped chromatin, frequent nucleoli, and many mitotic figures. Bizarre tumor giant cells and squamous metaplasia have been described (Figure 10.24). The loose connective tissue stroma between the sheets of tumor cells contains a diffuse, moderate to marked lymphoplasmacytic infiltrate. Finally, the tumor cells do not infiltrate the surrounding normal breast tissue, but rather the tumors have a circumscribed, pushing border (Figure 10.25). The presence of an in-situ component is rare but does not negate the diagnosis. Adjacent lobular units often show lymphocytic lobulitis.

When a usual NST component constitutes up to 25 percent of the tumor, and only mild to moderate lymphocytic infiltrate or focal margin infiltration is present (Figure 10.26), then the tumor may be classified as atypical medullary carcinoma to indicate that many features are present, but this is insufficient for a diagnosis of pure medullary carcinoma.

Medullary carcinomas are typically negative for hormone receptors and show no HER2/neu overexpression or gene amplification.

Differential Diagnosis

Strict adherence to diagnostic criteria is necessary when making a diagnosis of medullary carcinoma. Tumors showing less than 75 percent medullary component

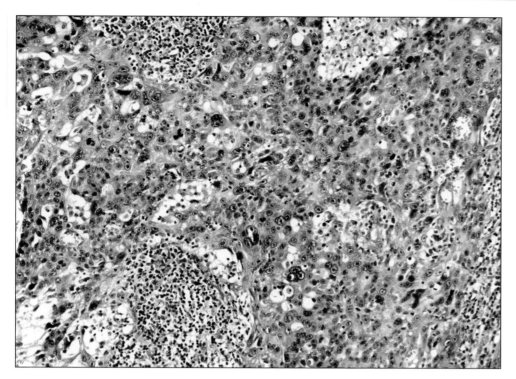

Figure 10.24. Medullary carcinoma. The tumor cells are large with pleomorphic nuclei, clumped chromatin, frequent nucleoli, and many mitotic figures. Bizarre tumor giant cells can be present.

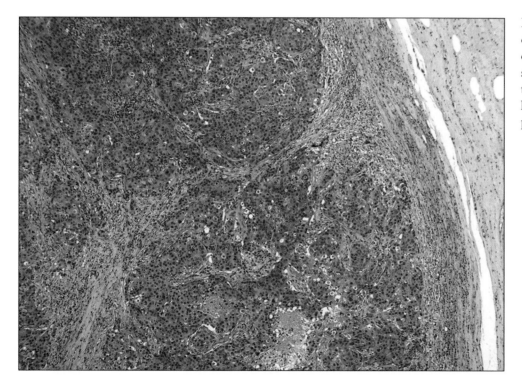

Figure 10.25. Medullary carcinoma. The tumor cells do not infiltrate the surrounding normal breast tissue, but rather the tumors have a circumscribed, pushing border.

should be classified as NST carcinoma, although the presence of medullary features may be mentioned in a comment. Many invasive carcinomas show a prominent lymphoplasmacytic infiltrate and its presence alone in the absence of other histologic features of medullary carcinoma is insufficient for establishing such a diagnosis.

Figure 10.26. Atypical medullary carcinoma. The morphology of the tumor is similar to medullary carcinoma, however, focal infiltration into the adjacent breast parenchyma is present.

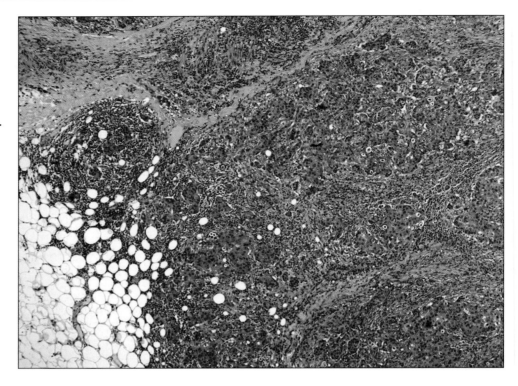

On rare occasions, in core biopsy material, metastatic carcinoma involving an intramammary or axillary lymph node may present diagnostic difficulties. Identification of residual lymph node structures, that is, subcapsular sinus, or the presence of germinal centers may help in this distinction.

Treatment and Prognosis

Regional lymph node metastases are present in about 23 percent of patients with medullary carcinoma. When strict histological criteria are used for diagnosis, node-negative medullary carcinoma predicts a good prognosis with five- and ten-year survival rates of 92 and 84 percent, respectively. In keeping with the high histologic grade and high proliferative activity of these tumors, recurrence and death usually occurs within 5 years after diagnosis. The predictive value of less extensive medullary features in carcinomas is not clear, although in node-negative cases it may be somewhat better compared to usual high-grade tumors.

Since medullary carcinomas and high-grade tumors with medullary features are more common among BRCA1-related cancers, such a diagnosis, especially in a young woman, should raise the possibility of genetic disposition.

INVASIVE PAPILLARY CARCINOMA

Clinical Features

Invasive papillary carcinomas are uncommon, accounting for less than 2 percent of all invasive breast cancers. Their incidence appears to be higher in postmenopausal women.

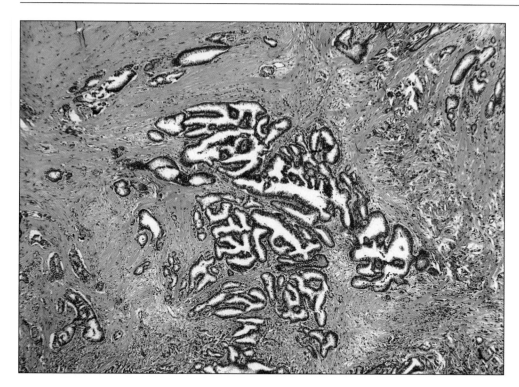

Figure 10.27. Invasive papillary carcinoma. The tumor is characterized by infiltrating islands of tumor cells lining fibrovascular cores.

Macroscopic and Microscopic Features

These tumors are usually small and have a variable gross appearance. They may be well circumscribed or present with macroscopic features indistinguishable from other breast carcinomas.

Microscopically, this special type is characterized by infiltrating islands of tumor cells lining fibrovascular cores (Figure 10.27). The papillary structures are usually more prominent at the periphery of the lesions, whereas other areas may be more closely packed and cellular, obscuring the papillary structures. The tumor cells have variable cytologic features and nuclear grade, and may show apocrine differentiation (Figure 10.28). Although no firm criteria have been defined, it was suggested that more than 90 percent of the tumor should show papillary features to be classified as an invasive papillary carcinoma. An associated in situ component, usually cribriform of papillary DCIS, is frequently present. ER and PR positivity, and HER2 negativity have been documented in this tumor type.

Differential Diagnosis

Invasive papillary carcinoma should be distinguished from invasive carcinomas arising in association with encapsulated (encysted or intracystic) papillary carcinomas, which are usually of no special type.

Given the rarity of invasive papillary carcinoma, a metastatic lesion from typical papillary carcinomas arising in other sites (e.g., thyroid or kidney) should always be considered. Identification of an in situ component favors a breast primary, whereas in cases of metastasis appropriate immunohistochemical stains and clinical history may aid in establishing a correct diagnosis.

Figure 10.28. Invasive papillary carcinoma. The tumor cells lining the papillary structures with fibrovascular cores may have variable cytologic features and nuclear grade.

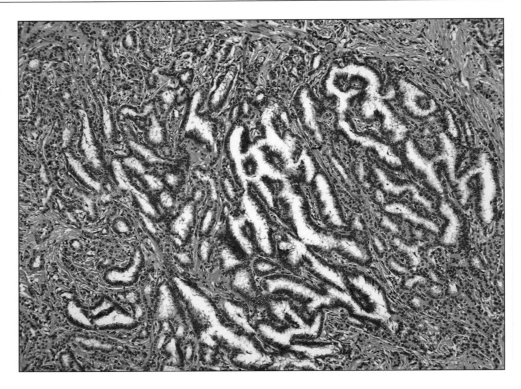

Treatment and Prognosis

Regional lymph node metastases have been reported in up to 32 percent of cases. In the reported series 80–90 percent five-year survival was found, which is comparable to other good prognosis special type carcinomas.

INVASIVE MICROPAPILLARY CARCINOMA

Invasive micropapillary carcinoma (IMPC) constitutes about 1.2–2.3 percent of all invasive breast cancers in its pure form, but it is much more frequently present (7 percent) as a component of mixed lesions. Although its histologic features have been well described in the literature and it is thought to represent the most inherently aggressive form of breast cancer, this special type is not well recognized in practice. IMPC has a special range of definition because its clinical importance is present even when it makes up only a small portion of the invasive component, which is in contrast with other special types of breast cancer that lose much of their prognostic significance if they do not represent the dominant pattern.

Clinical Features

The reported age of patients with IMPC at diagnosis ranges from 25 to 89 years with a median age of 52–62 years. Tumor size ranges from 0.3 to 10 cm (average 1.5 to 4.9 cm). Tumors with more than 50 percent micropapillary pattern tend to be larger

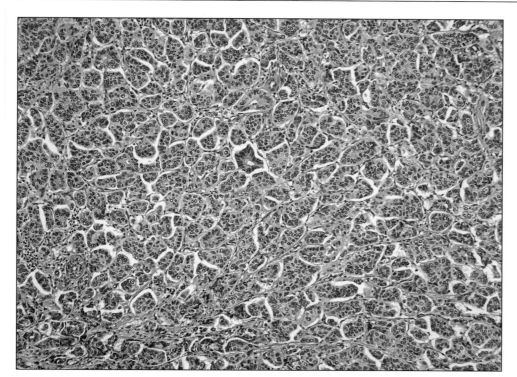

Figure 10.29. Invasive micropapillary carcinoma. These tumors show a characteristic infiltrating, nested pattern of tumor cells arranged in solid clusters or, less frequently, tubules.

and are diagnosed in older patients compared to tumors with only focal micropapillary features. The majority of the patients present with a palpable mass, but occasional lesions have been detected mammographically as a soft tissue density or as a result of microcalcifications.

Macroscopic and Microscopic Features

No distinguishing gross characteristics of IMPC have been described.

The characteristic histologic feature of IMPC is that of an infiltrating, nested pattern of tumor cells arranged in solid clusters or, less frequently, tubules (Figure 10.29). These micropapillae are of similar size and lack central fibrovascular cores. The cell clusters generally have serrated peripheral borders with a radial orientation from the center to the periphery of the group and they are separated from the surrounding dense fibrocollagenous or more delicate, reticular tissue by an apparent clear space. Although myxoid stroma has been described in a few cases, a desmoplastic stromal reaction is typically absent. The tumor cells are cuboidal to columnar with finely granular or dense, eosinophilic cytoplasm and intermediate to high-grade nuclei (Figure 10.30). Calcifications and psammoma bodies can be identified ranging from rare to numerous.

The characteristic clear spaces surrounding the tumor-cell nests of IMPC are not lined by endothelial cells, as also demonstrated by immunohistochemistry for vascular and lymphatic endothelial markers. Further, the clear spaces are usually not present on frozen sections of the tumors, suggesting that they most likely represent an unusual, but consistently present retraction artifact. Although the spaces usually appear to be empty on routine hematoxylin and eosin (H&E)

165

Figure 10.30. Invasive micropapillary carcinoma. The micropapillae are of similar size and lack central fibrovascular cores. The cell clusters generally have serrated peripheral borders with a radial orientation from the center to the periphery of the group and they are separated from the surrounding dense fibrocollagenous or more delicate, reticular tissue by an apparent clear space. The tumor cells are cuboidal to columnar with finely granular or dense, eosinophilic cytoplasm and intermediate- to high-grade nuclei.

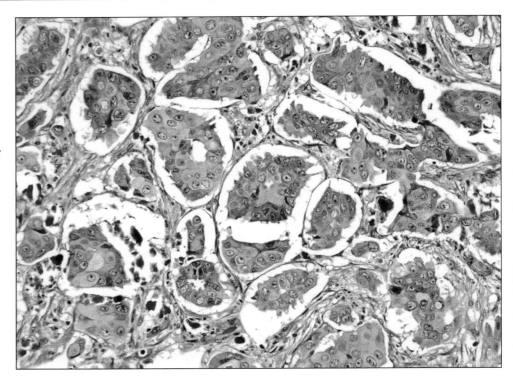

sections, mucinous material may be detectable by special stains in some cases. Indeed, a small subset (1–15 percent) of IMPC can show mucinous differentiation, however, the tumor cells in the mucin pools retain their characteristic micropapillary morphology (Figure 10.31).

Tumors with a pure micropapillary pattern are unusual. Rather, this critical histologic pattern is more frequently seen in association with common forms of NST carcinoma. Areas of carcinomas having IMPC growth pattern are typically identified at or near the infiltrating edge of the tumors and usually an abrupt transition is seen between usual and IMPC patterns, easily recognized at low magnification (Figure 10.32). In addition, the neoplastic cells in IMPC areas generally contain more abundant, eosinophilic cytoplasm compared to other areas of the tumors, also facilitating the recognition of this growth pattern.

The outer surface of the tumor cell clusters shows the presence of microvilli by electron microscopy and demonstrates histochemical and immunohistochemical features characteristic of luminal lining, such as immunoreactivity for EMA and MUC1 (Figure 10.33). These findings suggest that the tumor cells at the periphery of the clusters are oriented as though the clear spaces around them were glandular lumens. This characteristic growth pattern has been referred to as "inside out" as a defining feature of IMPC. However, true lumina may also be present in the center of the clusters suggesting that "bipolar" would also describe the peculiar polarity.

IMPC are positive for estrogen and progesterone receptors in 90 and 70 percent of cases, respectively, and more than half of the tumors were reported to be positive for HER2/neu. Molecular studies showed loss of heterozygosity in locus 17p13.1 (p53) in four of five cases of IMPC, with 80 percent concordance between molecular and immunohistochemical studies. None of the IMPCs studied was

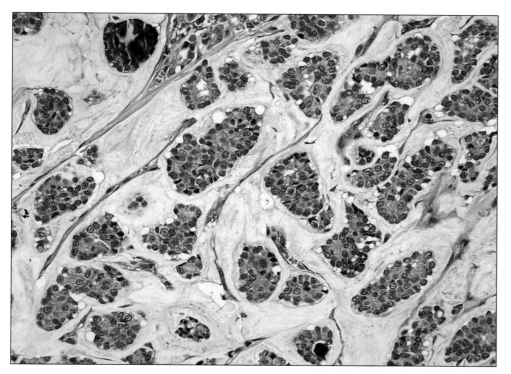

Figure 10.31. Invasive micropapillary carcinoma with mucinous features. A subset of invasive micropapillary carcinomas can show mucinous differentiation, however, the tumor cells in the mucin pools retain their characteristic micropapillary morphology.

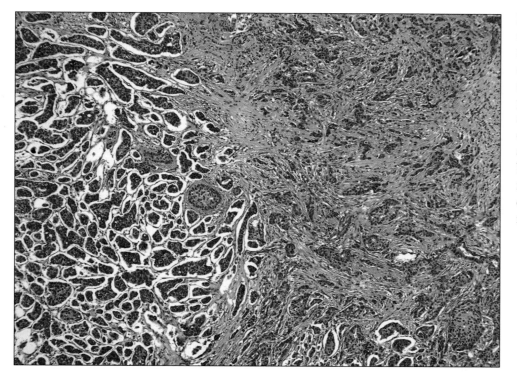

Figure 10.32. Invasive NST carcinoma with focal micropapillary features. Areas of carcinomas having micropapillary growth pattern are typically identified at or near the infiltrating edge of the tumors and usually an abrupt transition is seen between usual and micropapillary patterns, easily recognized at low magnification.

immunoreactive for basal cell markers, including CK5/6, EGFR, and c-kit. An important genetic feature of IMPC, identified by comparative genomic hybridization (CGH), appears to be the loss of genetic material from chromosome 8p, detected in 100 percent of cases examined.

Figure 10.33. Invasive micropapillary carcinoma. Immunohistochemical stain for epithelial membrane antigen highlights the characteristic "inside-out" or "bipolar" growth pattern of the tumors.

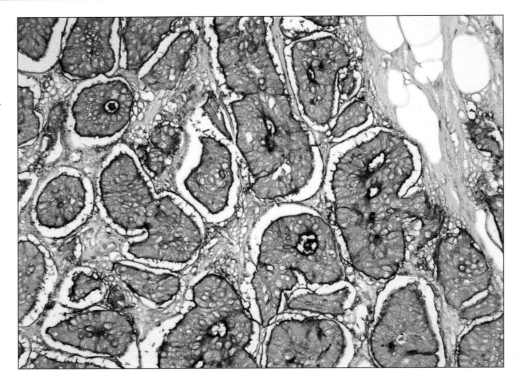

Differential Diagnosis

The differential diagnosis of IMPC includes mucinous carcinoma, invasive papillary carcinoma, extensive lymphovascular invasion, or extensive retraction artifact in usual NST carcinomas, and metastatic tumors involving the breast. The distinction from pure mucinous carcinoma is especially relevant, since mucin secretion can also be found in IMPC and the two patterns may coexist in some cases. Pure mucinous carcinoma features abundant pools of extracellular mucin that is absent from IMPC and the tumor clusters in mucinous carcinoma usually have smooth rather than serrated contours. Invasive papillary carcinoma lacks the clear spaces surrounding the tumor cell clusters, has a truly papillary architecture with fibrovascular cores, and typically shows low nuclear grade.

Extensive lymphatic invasion by NST carcinomas can also be confused with IMPC. Despite the similarity to lymphatic space involvement, the association of many such spaces clustered immediately adjacent to each other in IMPC denies that suggestion, as does the absence of endothelial lining. Since retraction artifact is present only within the invasive tumor mass, one should concentrate the search for foci of lymphovascular invasion to breast tissue outside the main tumor. However, lymphatic space involvement is often not equivocal in IMPC (Figure 10.34) and is best identified by using the localization of lymphatic channels in association with the venous and arterial clusters away from breast parenchymal elements. Extensive retraction artifact in usual NST carcinomas may also be confused with IMPC. One should also look for signs of the characteristic reverse polarity in IMPC, which feature can be highlighted with the use of special stains (EMA) when necessary.

Metastatic tumors, especially ovarian serous papillary carcinomas and less commonly, micropapillary variants of other carcinomas, that is, bladder and lung,

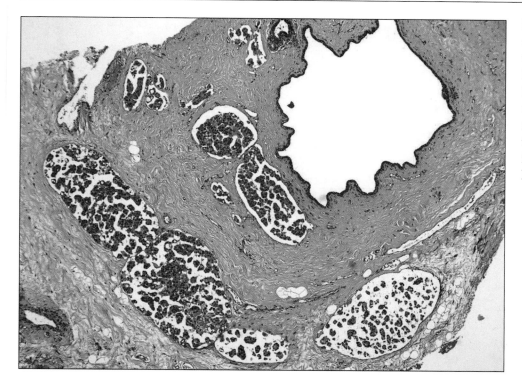

Figure 10.34. Invasive micropapillary carcinoma with extensive lymphovascular invasion. Note that the carcinoma retains its characteristic morphologic features within the lymphatic spaces as it does in metastatic deposits in lymph nodes or distant sites.

must also be considered in the differential diagnosis. Accurate clinical history, presence of an associated in-situ component and immunohistochemistry in occasional cases may aid in the diagnosis.

Treatment and Prognosis

Despite the small number of studies reported in the literature to date, IMPC pattern in breast carcinomas is undoubtedly not as rare as one would think. Recognition of this pattern, even as a small component of more ordinary breast carcinoma, is important, because it appears to be associated with meaningful clinical implications regardless of tumor size. There is consensus in the literature that IMPCs behave aggressively, with frequent lymphatic invasion and lymph node metastasis. Further, the high likelihood of (often extensive) lymphatic involvement appears to be operative even for tumors less than 1 cm in size, and when only a limited portion of the cancer has the micropapillary pattern. It is recommended that the presence of IMPC pattern should be mentioned in the pathology report with the relative percentage of the IMPC component.

Evaluation of regional lymph nodes is mandatory in cases of IMPC. Given the frequent and often extensive nodal involvement in these cases (up to 69–95 percent of reported cases), it was even suggested that patients with IMPC may not benefit from sentinel lymph node biopsy. Despite its propensity for multiple lymph node involvement, the outcome of IMPC patients does not appear to be different from that of NST carcinoma patients having similar lymph node status. Rather, the prognostic implications of IMPC are accounted for by the extent of lymphatic involvement and usual features relevant to prognosis and patient management, such as grade, hormone receptor status, and molecular markers.

Figure 10.35. Secretory carcinoma. The neoplastic cells are low grade and form microcystic spaces. The tumor cells have abundant amphophilic cytoplasm and contain intracystoplasmic secretory material.

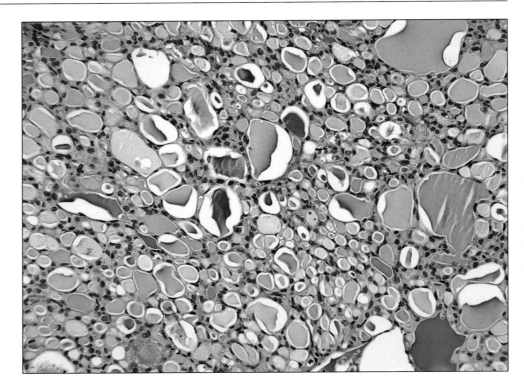

SECRETORY CARCINOMA

Secretory carcinoma is quite rare, accounting for less than 1 percent of all breast cancers. It was originally described in children by McDivitt and Stewart, who called it "juvenile carcinoma." However, approximately two-thirds of published cases occur in adults older than 20 years, and only one-third occur in children.

Clinical Features

Patients usually present with a small, well-circumscribed palpable mass, often near the areola. Patients present at a younger age overall compared to other types of breast cancer. Although most cases occur in women, it has been described in males as well.

Macroscopic and Microscopic Features

Grossly, secretory carcinomas tend to be well circumscribed with a gray/yellow cut surface. The mean tumor size is 1.6–2.6 cm.

Microscopically most tumors have a circumscribed border against the surrounding benign breast tissue. The neoplastic cells are low grade and form glands, microcystic, papillae, and solid nests (Figure 10.35). Mitoses are rare. The tumor cells have abundant clear or amphophilic cytoplasm, and focal apocrine differentiation may be seen. Tumors may be more cellular at the periphery of the lesions with central hyalinized areas. A characteristic histologic feature is the presence of abundant extra- and intracellular PAS-positive secretory material (Figure 10.36). In-situ disease of similar histologic features is often present.

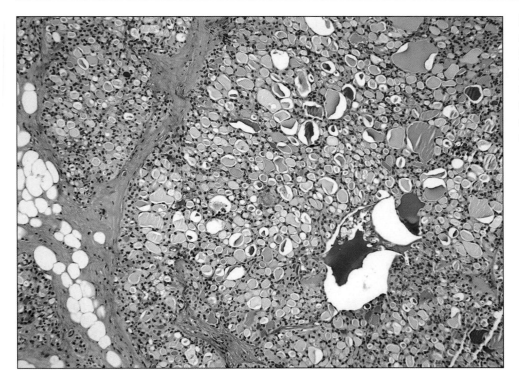

Figure 10.36. Secretory carcinoma. A characteristic histologic feature is the presence of abundant extra- and intracellular secretory material, which stains positively using PAS stain.

Hormone receptor expression is variable, although the majority of the tumors tend to be ER- and PR-negative, and show no HER2/neu overexpression. Strong immunoreactivity for S-100, α-lactalbumin, and polyclonal carcinoembryonic antigen (CEA) has been reported. Molecularly, secretory carcinomas show relatively low numbers of genetic alterations (2.0), however, they show the characteristic expression of the ETV6-NTRK3 fusion gene coding for a chimeric tyrosine kinase.

Differential Diagnosis

The main differential diagnosis of secretory carcinoma is with clear cell (lipid-rich and glycogen-rich) carcinomas. Tumors with these latter features show growth patterns of NST carcinomas and tend to be high combined histologic grade, in contrast with the circumscription, abundant extracellular secretory material, and low nuclear grade characteristic of secretory carcinoma.

Treatment and Prognosis

Despite the occasional presence of lymph node metastases, distant metastasis is unusual and the tumors are characterized by a favorable prognosis. The clinical course in both children and adults is characterized by a tendency for late local recurrence and prolonged survival even with lymph node metastasis, and death from metastatic tumor is exceedingly rare. However, some studies suggested a less favorable prognosis in adults and identified age less than 20 years, tumor size less than 2 cm, and absence of frank stromal invasion as markers of favorable prognosis.

Figure 10.37. Adenoid cystic carcinoma. The tumors are composed of nests made up of a dual population of neoplastic cells forming prominent crisp, "cribriform" spaces.

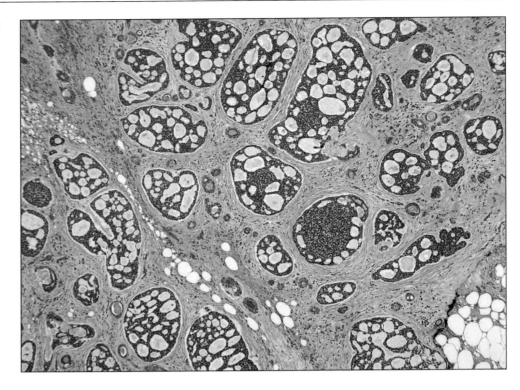

ADENOID CYSTIC CARCINOMA

ACC of the breast is very rare, representing about 0.1 percent of all breast cancers. Morphologically these tumors are similar to their counterparts arising in the salivary glands, but they are associated with an excellent prognosis.

Clinical Features

Patients with ACC tend to be postmenopausal in their sixties and seventies (the median age at presentation is 66 years). The tumors vary in size with an average diameter of 3 cm. The lesions may be painful and tend to occur in sub- or periareolar location.

Macroscopic and Microscopic Features

Grossly, the tumors appear to be well circumscribed. Because of the excellent prognostic implications of ACC, adherence to strict histologic criteria in its diagnosis is important. ACC is characteristically composed of a dual population of neoplastic cells (Figure 10.37). The main proliferating element has the appearance of vimentin-positive modified myoepithelial cells grouped in nests or outlining the characteristic cribriform spaces ("pseudolumens"), whereas cytokeratin- and EMA-positive epithelial cells line small ductule-like structures with true lumina (Figure 10.38). The cribriform spaces contain alcianophilic mucosubstances or amorphous eosinophilic basement membrane material, whereas the ductule-like structures contain PAS-positive material. PAS staining

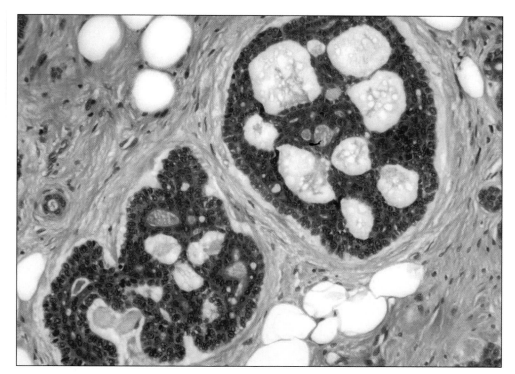

Figure 10.38. Adenoid cystic carcinoma. The dual cell population is evident at higher magnification. The predominant neoplastic element is composed of modified myoepithelial cells forming characteristic cribriform spaces containing alcianophilic mucosubstances. A second population of epithelial cells form ductule-like structures with true lumina containing PAS-positive material.

and collagen type IV immunostaining reveal a thick basal lamina bordering the cribriform structures but not the ductule-like structures. Occasionally, squamous metaplasia may be seen. An in-situ component may sometimes be present, particularly when the tumor is coexistent with microglandular adenosis. ACC is characteristically negative for hormone receptor expression and does not over-express HER2/neu.

Differential Diagnosis

NST breast carcinomas may show focal growth patterns reminiscent of ACC. Invasive cribriform carcinoma should also be considered in the differential diagnosis. In contrast with these tumors, the defining feature of ACC is the presence of two distinct types of neoplastic cells with the formation of two types of spaces. Immunohistochemical stains for myoepithelial (smooth muscle actin, S-100 protein, vimentin) and epithelial markers highlight these features. In contrast to invasive cribriform carcinoma, which is universally ER-positive, ACC is characteristically negative for ER.

Treatment and Prognosis

ACC of the breast is associated with an excellent prognosis. The incidence of axillary nodal metastases is very low, suggesting that nodal sampling may not be necessary in these cases. Local recurrence and distant metastasis are seen very rarely, although late recurrences (10–20 years) have been reported. A special feature of ACC is the frequent presence of extensive and grossly unapparent infiltration within the breast, which may necessitate reexcision or mastectomy to achieve negative margins.

Although efforts have been made to grade ACC using a system similar to that applied for salivary gland tumors, histologic grade does not appear to predict biologic behavior of ACC of the breast.

RARE HISTOLOGIC PATTERNS OF INVASIVE CARCINOMA

This section discusses rare patterns of invasive carcinoma that are generally identified by single features. Although some of these entities have been proposed as special types of breast cancer, the presence of the characteristic features do not provide any clinical or prognostic relevance beyond that of combined histologic grade and thus, at present they are not regarded as specific diagnostic entities. As mentioned in the previous discussion, reporting the presence of these features in otherwise NST carcinomas is only relevant to acknowledge that they have been recognized and that they may also be present in later metastases.

Invasive Carcinoma with Apocrine Features

Focal apocrine differentiation is quite common in breast carcinomas; it has been reported in up to 60 percent of NST carcinomas and also in special type carcinomas such as papillary, micropapillary, and lobular carcinomas. It was suggested that more than 90 percent of the cancer cells should show apocrine cytologic features to be classified as apocrine carcinoma. Despite this recommendation, the reported incidence of pure invasive apocrine carcinoma is 0.3–4 percent in the literature, likely reflecting differences in diagnostic criteria.

Apocrine carcinomas present as mass lesions without any characteristic clinical or radiologic features. Grossly, these tumors are indistinguishable from other mammary carcinomas and usually present as firm to hard masses with infiltrating borders. Similarly, tumor size, grade, and incidence of lymph node positivity are not significantly different from NST carcinomas.

Microscopically, apocrine carcinomas show similar architectural patterns as other NST carcinomas, and differ only in the cytologic appearance of the constituent cells (Figure 10.39). The tumor cells are characterized by abundant eosinophilic, granular, foamy or clear cytoplasm and round nuclei with prominent, and often multiple, nucleoli (Figure 10.40).

Immunohistochemically, apocrine carcinomas tend to be ER- and PR-negative, but usually show strong expression of androgen receptor (AR). However, AR positivity is not restricted to apocrine carcinomas as it is present in up to 60 percent of NST carcinomas as well. HER2/neu overexpression and/or gene amplification in apocrine carcinomas has been reported in up to 50 percent of the cases. The cytoplasm of tumor cells stain strongly for gross cystic disease fluid protein-15 (GCDFP-15) by immunohistochemistry.

Apocrine carcinomas may be mimicked by benign lesions such as sclerosing adenosis with apocrine change (apocrine adenosis), especially if the cells show cytologic atypia. Recognition of the underlying lobular architecture of sclerosing adenosis (best appreciated at low power) and the use of immunohistochemical stains for myoepithelial markers can help in establishing a correct diagnosis.

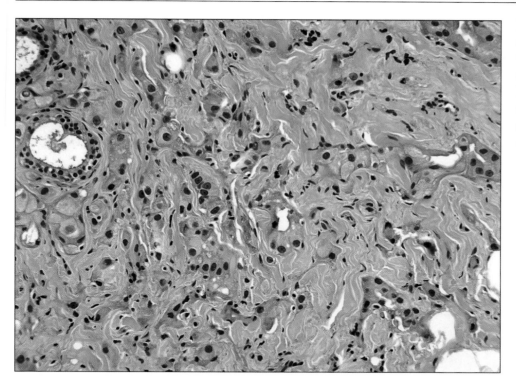

Figure 10.39. Invasive apocrine carcinoma. These tumors show similar architectural patterns to other NST carcinomas, and differ only in the apocrine cytologic appearance of the constituent cells.

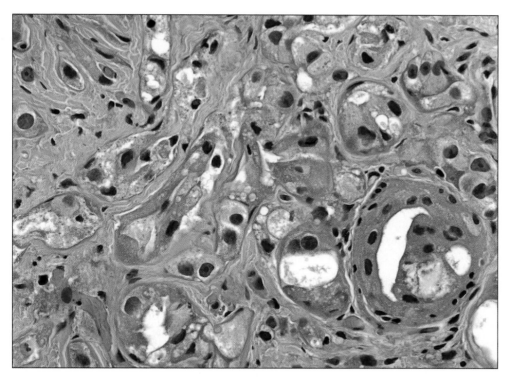

Figure 10.40. Invasive apocrine carcinoma. The tumor cells are characterized by abundant eosinophilic, granular, foamy, or clear cytoplasm often containing apocrine granules. The nuclei are round with prominent, and often multiple, nucleoli.

Studies addressing the clinical significance of apocrine differentiation in breast carcinomas showed no significant differences when compared to matched cohorts of NST tumors and concluded that apocrine carcinoma is not clinically distinct from NST carcinomas. Although there is currently insufficient evidence

Figure 10.41. Invasive carcinoma with clear cell (glycogen-rich) features. The tumors have the architectural features of NST carcinomas, but the constituent cells have abundant clear cytoplasm with a centrally placed nucleus.

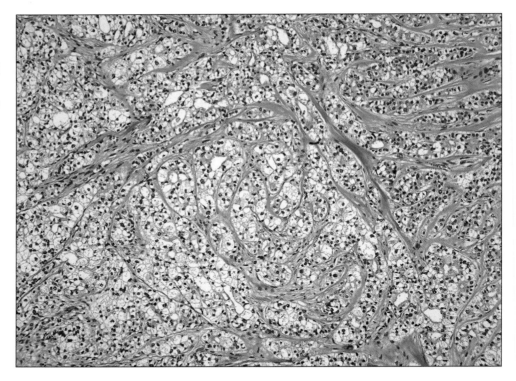

to recognize the apocrine phenotype as a special type carcinoma, this feature should be mentioned in the pathology report when prominent. Further studies are needed to explore the potential utility of antiandrogenic therapy in breast cancers showing AR expression.

Invasive Carcinomas with Clear Cell (Glycogen-Rich and Lipid-Rich) Features

Clear cytoplasm in invasive breast carcinomas may be due to various factors, including artifacts of tissue fixation. Abundant intracytoplasmic glycogen as a basis for clear cell change is relatively uncommon in breast cancers (glycogen-rich breast carcinomas). The tumors have the architectural features of NST carcinomas, but the constituent cells have abundant clear cytoplasm with a centrally placed nucleus (Figure 10.41). Apocrine features may also be present; in fact, it was suggested that these tumors may represent a variant of apocrine carcinoma. Intracytoplasmic glycogen may be demonstrated by diastase-labile PAS positivity. Although the presence of tumor cells with clear cytoplasm is not associated with any particular subtype of breast cancer, these tumors tend to have high-grade nuclei and are of high combined histologic grade. Although clear cell change, which is also found in a variety of benign breast lesions, is not associated with any clinical or prognostic significance other than that provided by histologic grade and tumor stage, the finding of a clear cell neoplasm in the breast should raise the possibility of a metastasis from a traditionally clear cell tumor, for example, renal cell carcinoma, and must be ruled out.

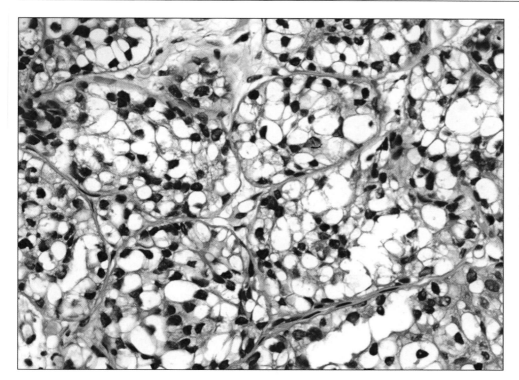

Figure 10.42. Invasive carcinoma with clear cell (lipid-rich) features. The architectural pattern is similar to usual NST carcinomas, but the tumors tend to be poorly differentiated without gland formation and show prominent nuclear atypia. The constituent cells have abundant foamy, vacuolated cytoplasm containing neutral lipid.

The presence of tumor cells with foamy, vacuolated, lipid-rich cytoplasm is not associated with any particular subtype of breast cancer. The tumor cells contain neutral lipid, which can be highlighted using special stains such as oil red O or Sudan black. The architectural pattern is similar to usual NST carcinomas, but tends to be poorly differentiated without gland formation. Nuclear atypia is usually prominent, and thus, breast cancers composed of tumor cells with lipid-rich cytoplasm are usually of high combined histologic grade (Figure 10.42). There is currently no evidence that the presence of cytoplasmic neutral lipid has any clinical or prognostic implication in addition to that recognized by histologic grade.

Invasive Carcinoma with Signet-Ring Cell Features

Signet-ring cells are found in a wide variety of both malignant and benign breast lesions. Breast carcinomas, in particular lobular carcinomas, have a tendency to feature prominent signet-ring cells in association with high nuclear grade (Figure 10.43). The presence of signet-ring cells has no specific clinical or prognostic importance, and the apparent poor prognosis attributed to signet-ring cell carcinomas in some studies is most likely related to high tumor grade. Nevertheless, commenting on the presence of prominent signet-ring cell features in breast cancers is important, because later metastases to organs in which signet-ring cell carcinomas may arise can be mistaken for a primary lesion. In such cases, immunohistochemical stains for CDX2, GCDFP-15, hormone receptors, and cytokeratins 7 and 20 may aid in the diagnosis.

Figure 10.43. Invasive carcinoma with signet-ring cell features. The tumor cells contain intracytoplasmic mucin, which pushes the nuclei to the side. This cytologic feature tends to be associated with high nuclear grade in breast cancers.

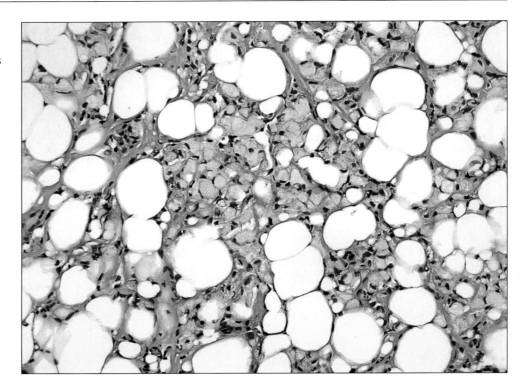

Invasive Carcinomas with Neuroendocrine Features

Focal neuroendocrine differentiation, assessed by immunohistochemical positivity for neuroendocrine markers, is relatively common in breast carcinomas (10–20 percent), and does not appear to have any prognostic or clinical implication.

Primary small cell carcinoma of the breast is very rare with approximately ten cases reported in the literature. Age at presentation varies from 41 to 69 years. Grossly, the tumors measure an average of 3 cm in size and demonstrate irregular borders. Microscopically these tumors are similar to small cell carcinomas arising in other organs, such as lung. An in-situ component, composed of similar cells, can be present. Lymphovascular invasion is frequent and most patients have lymph node metastases at the time of diagnosis. Immunohistochemical stains are positive for cytokeratins and neuroendocrine markers, such as neuron specific enolase (NSE), CD56, chromogranin, and synaptophysin. Small cell carcinomas are usually negative for ER and PR expression. The differential diagnosis is metastatic small cell carcinoma arising in another organ, usually lung, and this possibility should be rigorously ruled out before accepting the tumor as a breast primary. This can be done mostly by clinical means as TTF-1 positivity was reported in 20 percent of small cell carcinomas of the breast. Identification of an in-situ component and CK7 positivity favors a breast primary. Although small cell carcinoma of the breast is reported to have a poor prognosis with most cases being fatal, this may be due to associated other prognostic features such as high combined histologic grade, frequent lymph node involvement and lack of ER expression.

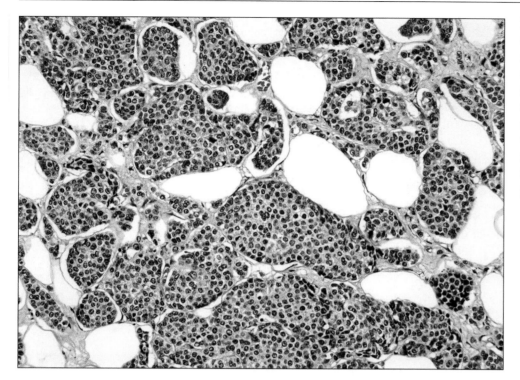

Figure 10.44. Invasive carcinoma with neuroendocrine features (carcinoid pattern). The tumor cells are arranged in nests, cords, and acini. The constituent cells are uniform with scant cytoplasm, uniform round nuclei, and finely granular chromatin pattern.

Lower grade invasive breast carcinomas with neuroendocrine features are similar to carcinoid tumors found elsewhere in the body. These tumors present as firm, rubbery masses ranging in size from 1 to 4 cm. Grossly, they show a solid, homogenous cut surface. Microscopically, the tumor cells are arranged in nests, cords, and acini. The cells are uniform with scant cytoplasm, uniform round nuclei, and finely granular chromatin pattern (Figure 10.44). Immuno-histochemically, the tumors show diffuse positivity for neuroendocrine markers. The presence of dense core granules can be confirmed by electron microscopy. The most important differential diagnosis is with metastatic carcinoid tumor from a primary in another organ, usually the gastrointestinal tract. Appropriate history and clinical examination are important in making this distinction. These tumors may also be confused with some in-situ and invasive lobular carcinomas, especially with the alveolar variant. Breast carcinomas with carcinoid pattern do not appear to be associated with specific clinical or prognostic implications, other than standard prognostic features such as grade and stage.

REFERENCES

Invasive Lobular Carcinoma

Acs G, Lawton TJ, Rebbeck TR, et al. Differential expression of E-cadherin in lobular and ductal neoplasms of the breast and its biologic and diagnostic implications. *Am J Clin Pathol.* 2001;115:85–98.

Da SL, Parry S, Reid L, et al. Aberrant expression of E-cadherin in lobular carcinomas of the breast. *Am J Surg Pathol.* 2008;32:773–83.

DiCostanzo D, Rosen PP, Gareen I, et al. Prognosis in infiltrating lobular carcinoma: an analysis of "classical" and variant tumors. *Am J Surg Pathol.* 1990;14:12–23.

Dixon JM, Anderson TJ, Page DL, et al. Infiltrating lobular carcinoma of the breast. *Histopathology.* 1982;6:149–61.

Eusebi V, Magalhaes F, Azzopardi JG. Pleomorphic lobular carcinoma of the breast: an aggressive tumor showing apocrine differentiation. *Hum Pathol.* 1992;23:655–62.

Fechner RE. Histologic variants of infiltrating lobular carcinoma of the breast. *Hum Pathol.* 1975;6:373–8.

Martinez V, Azzopardi JG. Invasive lobular carcinoma of the breast: incidence and variants. *Histopathology.* 1979;3:467–88.

Page DL, Anderson TJ, Sakamoto G. Infiltrating carcinoma: major histologic types. In: Page DL, Anderson TJ, eds. *Diagnostic Histopathology of the Breast.* London: WB Saunders; 193–235.

Pestalozzi BC, Zahrieh D, Mallon E, et al. Distinct clinical and prognostic features of infiltrating lobular carcinoma of the breast: combined results of 15 International Breast Cancer Study Group clinical trials. *J Clin Oncol.* 2008;26:3006–14.

Pinder SE, Elston CW, Ellis IO. Invasive carcinoma – usual histologic types. In: Elston CW, Ellis IO, eds. *The Breast.* Edinburgh: Churchill Livingstone; 1998;283–337.

Reis-Filho JS, Simpson PT, Jones C, et al. Pleomorphic lobular carcinoma of the breast: role of comprehensive molecular pathology in characterization of an entity. *J Pathol.* 2005; 207:1–13.

Sastre-Garau X, Jouve M, Asselain B, et al. Infiltrating lobular carcinoma of the breast. Clinicopathologic analysis of 975 cases with reference to data on conservative therapy and metastatic patterns. *Cancer.* 1996;77:113–20.

Tot T. The diffuse type of invasive lobular carcinoma of the breast: morphology and prognosis. *Virchows Arch.* 2003;443:718–24.

Weidner N, Semple JP. Pleomorphic variant of invasive lobular carcinoma of the breast. *Hum Pathol.* 1992;23:1167–71.

Wheeler JE, Enterline HT. Lobular carcinoma of the breast in situ and infiltrating. *Pathol Annu.* 1976;11:161–88.

Tubular Carcinoma

Abdel-Fatah TM, Powe DG, Hodi Z, et al. High frequency of coexistence of columnar cell lesions, lobular neoplasia, and low grade ductal carcinoma in situ with invasive tubular carcinoma and invasive lobular carcinoma. *Am J Surg Pathol.* 2007;31:417–26.

Cserni G, Bianchi S, Vezzosi V, et al. Sentinel lymph node biopsy and non-sentinel node involvement in special type breast carcinomas with a good prognosis. *Eur J Cancer.* 2007;43:1407–14.

Deos PH, Norris HJ. Well-differentiated (tubular) carcinoma of the breast: a clinicopathologic study of 145 pure and mixed cases. *Am J Clin Pathol.* 1982;78:1–7.

Diab SG, Clark GM, Osborne CK, et al. Tumor characteristics and clinical outcome of tubular and mucinous breast carcinomas. *J Clin Oncol.* 1999;17:1442–8.

McDivitt RW, Boyce W, Gersell D. Tubular carcinoma of the breast. Clinical and pathological observations concerning 135 cases. *Am J Surg Pathol.* 1982;6:401–11.

Oberman HA, Fidler WJ, Jr. Tubular carcinoma of the breast. *Am J Surg Pathol.* 1979;3: 387–95.

Sullivan T, Raad RA, Goldberg S, et al. Tubular carcinoma of the breast: a retrospective analysis and review of the literature. *Breast Cancer Res Treat.* 2005;93:199–205.

Waldman FM, Hwang ES, Etzell J, et al. Genomic alterations in tubular breast carcinomas. *Hum Pathol.* 2001;32:222–6.

Invasive Cribriform Carcinoma

Page DL, Dixon JM, Anderson TJ, et al. Invasive cribriform carcinoma of the breast. *Histopathology.* 1983;7:525–36.
Venable JG, Schwartz AM, Silverberg SG. Infiltrating cribriform carcinoma of the breast: a distinctive clinicopathologic entity. *Hum Pathol.* 1990;21:333–8.

Tubulolobular Carcinoma

Esposito NN, Chivukula M, Dabbs DJ. The ductal phenotypic expression of the E-cadherin/catenin complex in tubulolobular carcinoma of the breast: an immunohistochemical and clinicopathologic study. *Mod Pathol.* 2007;20:130–8.
Fisher ER, Gregorio RM, Redmond C, et al. Tubulolobular invasive breast cancer: a variant of lobular invasive cancer. *Hum Pathol.* 1977;8:679–83.
Green I, McCormick B, Cranor M, et al. A comparative study of pure tubular and tubulolobular carcinoma of the breast. *Am J Surg Pathol.* 1997;21:653–7.
Wheeler DT, Tai LH, Bratthauer GL, et al. Tubulolobular carcinoma of the breast: an analysis of 27 cases of a tumor with a hybrid morphology and immunoprofile. *Am J Surg Pathol.* 2004;28:1587–93.

Mucinous Carcinoma

Clayton F. Pure mucinous carcinomas of breast: morphologic features and prognostic correlates. *Hum Pathol.* 1986;17:34–8.
Komaki K, Sakamoto G, Sugano H, et al. Mucinous carcinoma of the breast in Japan. A prognostic analysis based on morphologic features. *Cancer.* 1988;61:989–96.
Rasmussen BB. Human mucinous breast carcinomas and their lymph node metastases: a histological review of 247 cases. *Pathol Res Pract.* 1985;180:377–82.
Rasmussen BB, Rose C, Christensen IB. Prognostic factors in primary mucinous breast carcinoma. *Am J Clin Pathol.* 1987;87:155–60.

Medullary Carcinoma

Bloom HJ, Richardson WW, Field JR. Host resistance and survival in carcinoma of breast: a study of 104 cases of medullary carcinoma in a series of 1,411 cases of breast cancer followed for 20 years. *Br Med J.* 1970;3:181–8.
Moore OS, Jr., Foote FW, Jr. The relatively favorable prognosis of medullary carcinoma of the breast. *Cancer.* 1949;2:635–42.
Pedersen L, Holck S, Schiodt T. Medullary carcinoma of the breast. *Cancer Treat Rev.* 1988;15:53–63.
Pedersen L, Holck S, Schiodt T, et al. Medullary carcinoma of the breast, prognostic importance of characteristic histopathological features evaluated in a multivariate Cox analysis. *Eur J Cancer.* 1994;30A:1792–7.

Ridolfi RL, Rosen PP, Port A, et al. Medullary carcinoma of the breast: a clinicopathologic study with 10 year follow-up. *Cancer.* 1977;40:1365–85.

Shousha S. Medullary carcinoma of the breast and BRCA1 mutation. *Histopathology.* 2000;37:182–5.

Wargotz ES, Silverberg SG. Medullary carcinoma of the breast: a clinicopathologic study with appraisal of current diagnostic criteria. *Hum Pathol.* 1988;19:1340–6.

Invasive Papillary Carcinoma

Fisher ER, Palekar AS, Redmond C, et al. Pathologic findings from the National Surgical Adjuvant Breast Project (protocol no. 4). VI. Invasive papillary cancer. *Am J Clin Pathol.* 1980;73:313–22.

Invasive Micropapillary Carcinoma

Luna-More S, de los SF, Breton JJ, et al. Estrogen and progesterone receptors, c-erbB-2, p53, and Bcl-2 in thirty-three invasive micropapillary breast carcinomas. *Pathol Res Pract.* 1996;192:27–32.

Luna-More S, Gonzalez B, Acedo C, et al. Invasive micropapillary carcinoma of the breast. A new special type of invasive mammary carcinoma. *Pathol Res Pract.* 1994;190:668–74.

Middleton LP, Tressera F, Sobel ME, et al. Infiltrating micropapillary carcinoma of the breast. *Mod Pathol.* 1999;12:499–504.

Nassar H, Wallis T, Andea A, et al. Clinicopathologic analysis of invasive micropapillary differentiation in breast carcinoma. *Mod Pathol.* 2001;14:836–41.

Pettinato G, Manivel CJ, Panico L, et al. Invasive micropapillary carcinoma of the breast: clinicopathologic study of 62 cases of a poorly recognized variant with highly aggressive behavior. *Am J Clin Pathol.* 2004;121:857–66.

Siriaunkgul S, Tavassoli FA. Invasive micropapillary carcinoma of the breast. *Mod Pathol.* 1993;6:660–2.

Thor AD, Eng C, Devries S, et al. Invasive micropapillary carcinoma of the breast is associated with chromosome 8 abnormalities detected by comparative genomic hybridization. *Hum Pathol.* 2002;33:628–31.

Walsh MM, Bleiweiss IJ. Invasive micropapillary carcinoma of the breast: eighty cases of an underrecognized entity. *Hum Pathol.* 2001;32:583–9.

Zekioglu O, Erhan Y, Ciris M, et al. Invasive micropapillary carcinoma of the breast: high incidence of lymph node metastasis with extranodal extension and its immunohistochemical profile compared with invasive ductal carcinoma. *Histopathology.* 2004;44:18–23.

Secretory Carcinoma

Diallo R, Tognon C, Knezevich SR, et al. Secretory carcinoma of the breast: a genetically defined carcinoma entity. *Verh Dtsch Ges Pathol.* 2003;87:193–203.

Krausz T, Jenkins D, Grontoft O, et al. Secretory carcinoma of the breast in adults: emphasis on late recurrence and metastasis. *Histopathology.* 1989;14:25–36.

McDivitt RW, Stewart FW. Breast carcinoma in children. *JAMA.* 1966;195:388–90.

Oberman HA. Secretory carcinoma of the breast in adults. *Am J Surg Pathol.* 1980;4:465–70.

Rosen PP, Cranor ML. Secretory carcinoma of the breast. *Arch Pathol Lab Med.* 1991;115:141–4.

Tavassoli FA, Norris HJ. Secretory carcinoma of the breast. *Cancer.* 1980;45:2404–13.

Adenoid Cystic Carcinoma

Acs G, Simpson JF, Bleiweiss IJ, et al. Microglandular adenosis with transition into adenoid cystic carcinoma of the breast. *Am J Surg Pathol.* 2003;27:1052–60.

Anthony PP, James PD. Adenoid cystic carcinoma of the breast: prevalence, diagnostic criteria, and histogenesis. *J Clin Pathol.* 1975;28:647–55.

Kasami M, Olson SJ, Simpson JF, et al. Maintenance of polarity and a dual cell population in adenoid cystic carcinoma of the breast: an immunohistochemical study. *Histopathology.* 1998;32:232–8.

Lamovec J, Us-Krasovec M, Zidar A, et al. Adenoid cystic carcinoma of the breast: a histologic, cytologic, and immunohistochemical study. *Semin Diagn Pathol.* 1989;6:153–64.

Peters GN, Wolff M. Adenoid cystic carcinoma of the breast. Report of 11 new cases: review of the literature and discussion of biological behavior. *Cancer.* 1983;52:680–6.

Ro JY, Silva EG, Gallager HS. Adenoid cystic carcinoma of the breast. *Hum Pathol.* 1987;18:1276–81.

Rare Histologic Patterns of Invasive Carcinoma

Abati AD, Kimmel M, Rosen PP. Apocrine mammary carcinoma: a clinicopathologic study of 72 cases. *Am J Clin Pathol.* 1990;94:371–7.

Eusebi V, Magalhaes F, Azzopardi JG. Pleomorphic lobular carcinoma of the breast: an aggressive tumor showing apocrine differentiation. *Hum Pathol.* 1992;23:655–62.

Eusebi V, Millis RR, Cattani MG, et al. Apocrine carcinoma of the breast: a morphologic and immunocytochemical study. *Am J Pathol.* 1986;123:532–41.

Fisher ER, Tavares J, Bulatao IS, et al. Glycogen-rich, clear cell breast cancer: with comments concerning other clear cell variants. *Hum Pathol.* 1985;16:1085–90.

Fp, Bane A. An update on apocrine lesions of the breast. *Histopathology.* 2008;52:3–10.

Fp, Bane AL. The spectrum of apocrine lesions of the breast. *Adv Anat Pathol.* 2004;11:1–9.

Hayes MM, Seidman JD, Ashton MA. Glycogen-rich clear cell carcinoma of the breast: a clinicopathologic study of 21 cases. *Am J Surg Pathol.* 1995;19:904–11.

Hull MT, Seo IS, Battersby JS, et al. Signet-ring cell carcinoma of the breast: a clinico-pathologic study of 24 cases. *Am J Clin Pathol.*1980;73:31–5.

Hull MT, Warfel KA. Glycogen-rich clear cell carcinomas of the breast: a clinicopathologic and ultrastructural study. *Am J Surg Pathol.* 1986;10:553–9.

Kondo Y, Akita T, Sugano I, et al. Signet ring cell carcinoma of the breast. *Acta Pathol Jpn.* 1984;34:875–80.

Mazzella FM, Sieber SC, Braza F. Ductal carcinoma of male breast with prominent lipid-rich component. *Pathology.* 1995;27:280–3.

Merino MJ, LiVolsi VA. Signet ring carcinoma of the female breast: a clinicopathologic analysis of 24 cases. *Cancer.* 1981;48:1830–7.

Miremadi A, Pinder SE, Lee AH, et al. Neuroendocrine differentiation and prognosis in breast adenocarcinoma. *Histopathology.* 2002;40:215–22.

Papotti M, Gherardi G, Eusebi V, et al. Primary oat cell (neuroendocrine) carcinoma of the breast: report of four cases. *Virchows Arch A Pathol Anat Histopathol.* 1992;420:103–8.

Papotti M, Macri L, Finzi G, et al. Neuroendocrine differentiation in carcinomas of the breast: a study of 51 cases. *Semin Diagn Pathol.* 1989;6:174–88.

Ramos CV, Taylor HB. Lipid-rich carcinoma of the breast: a clinicopathologic analysis of 13 examples. *Cancer.* 1974;33:812–19.

Sapino A, Righi L, Cassoni P, et al. Expression of the neuroendocrine phenotype in carcinomas of the breast. *Semin Diagn Pathol.* 2000;17:127–37.

Van Krimpen C, Elferink A, Broodman CA, et al. The prognostic influence of neuroendocrine differentiation in breast cancer: results of a long-term follow-up study. *Breast.* 2004;13:329–33.

Van Laarhoven HA, Gratama S, Wereldsma JC. Neuroendocrine carcinoid tumours of the breast: a variant of carcinoma with neuroendocrine differentiation. *J Surg Oncol.* 1991;46:125–32.

Wade PM, Jr., Mills SE, Read M, et al. Small cell neuroendocrine (oat cell) carcinoma of the breast. *Cancer.* 1983;52:121–5.

Wrba F, Ellinger A, Reiner G, et al. Ultrastructural and immunohistochemical characteristics of lipid-rich carcinoma of the breast. *Virchows Arch A Pathol Anat Histopathol.* 1988;413:381–5.

11 INVASIVE CARCINOMA, NO SPECIAL TYPE

Thomas J. Lawton, MD

General Features and Histology/Grading	185
Prognostic and Predictive Factors	187
Invasive Carcinoma with Basal Phenotype	196

GENERAL FEATURES AND HISTOLOGY/GRADING

Invasive mammary carcinoma, no special type (NST) accounts for approximately 65–75 percent of invasive carcinomas of the breast. Although the term invasive ductal carcinoma has been used for this type of carcinoma, since many of the tumors do not form ducts, we feel this categorization is best used to separate out the majority of invasive carcinomas that cannot be placed into a special type category.

Invasive mammary carcinoma, NST, can present as a palpable mass or an incidental finding on breast imaging. A common gross appearance of these carcinomas is that of a sclerotic, stellate mass (Figure 11.1); however, some tumors appear well-circumscribed. The size of these tumors varies widely from several millimeters to greater than 10 cm.

Invasive mammary carcinoma, NST, is graded most commonly using the Nottingham system (modified Scarff-Bloom-Richardson scheme). In this system, tumors are graded on a scale of I–III, with grade I being well differentiated and grade III being poorly differentiated. The tumors are each scored on three variables, each given a score of 1–3: amount of tubule formation, nuclear grade, and mitotic rate. Tubule formation is graded as follows: a score of 1 for tumors with >75 percent tubule formation (Figure 11.2A); a score of 2 for tumors with 10–75 percent tubule formation (Figure 11.2B); and a score of 3 for tumors with <10 percent tubule formation (Figure11.2C). Nuclear grade is somewhat more subjective. A score of 1 is for nuclei that resemble those of normal ductal epithelium – the cells are small, generally round, and lack appreciable pleomorphism or nucleolation (Figure 11.3A); a score of 2 is for nuclei that show moderate pleomorphism and may have nucleoli appreciable at lower power (Figure 11.3B); and a score of 3 is for nuclei that show marked pleomorphism, generally with easily recognized nucleoli (Figure 11.3C). Mitotic activity is scored based on the number of mitotic figures present in 10 hpfs (field diameters vary among microscopes and standardization is recommended when counting mitotic figures). Mitotic figures should be clearly identified

Figure 11.1. Gross appearance of a typical invasive ductal carcinoma showing a sclerotic, white tumor with a stellate configuration within the fatty background of the breast tissue.

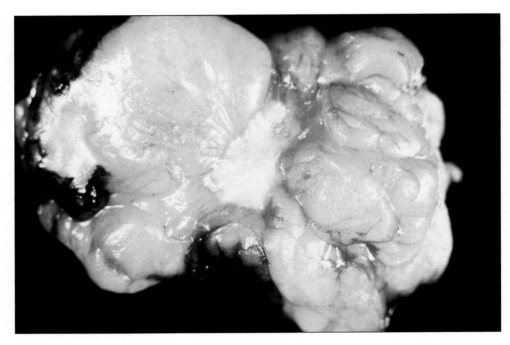

Figure 11.2. (A) Good tubule formation in an invasive carcinoma, NST. Note the vast majority of the tumor is composed of open tubules (>75 percent).
(B) Intermediate tubule formation in an invasive carcinoma, NST. In this case, most of the tumor is composed of nests and trabeculae with less open tubule formation (10–75 percent). (C) Poor tubule formation in an invasive carcinoma, NST. In this case, the tumor is composed of solid nests of cells with no tubule formation.

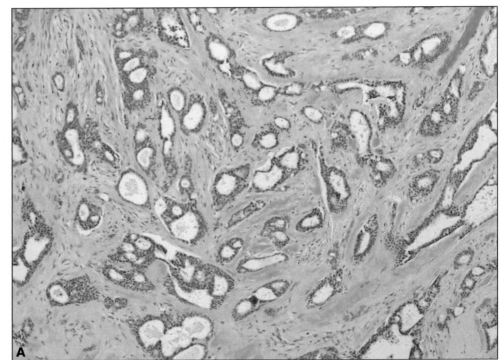

and pyknotic cells should not be counted (Figure 11.4). Proper fixation can greatly assist in the accurate counting of mitotic activity. The advancing edge of the invasive carcinoma is where the mitotic rate is preferably counted. The aforementioned scores are then added and the grade is assigned as follows: a score of 3–5 = grade I, a score of 6–7 = grade II, and a score of 8–9 = grade III.

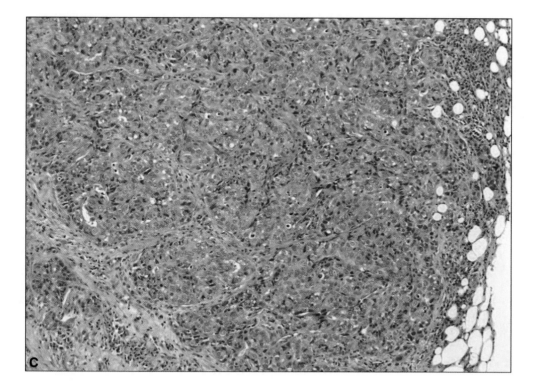

Figure 11.2. *(continued)*

PROGNOSTIC AND PREDICTIVE FACTORS

Lymph node status remains the most important independent prognostic marker for invasive carcinoma. With the advent of sentinel node biopsy and the

Figure 11.3. (A) Low nuclear grade in an invasive carcinoma, NST. The cells are small, with relatively uniform nuclei without nuclear pleomorphism. (B) Intermediate nuclear grade in an invasive carcinoma, NST. Here, the cells are larger, many with small nucleoli but no significant pleomorphism is noted. (C) High nuclear grade in an invasive carcinoma, NST. Note the marked pleomorphism of the cells with prominent nucleoli.

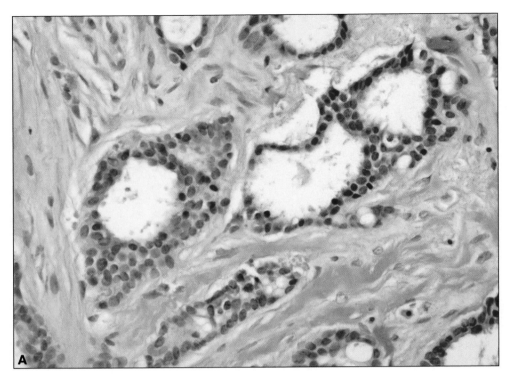

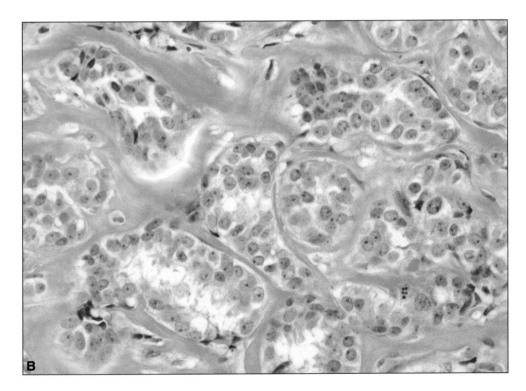

associated use of immunohistochemistry, changes have been made to the staging system for lymph node involvement. Macrometastases are tumor deposits greater than 2 mm. Micrometastases are defined as tumor deposits measuring less than 2 mm but greater than 0.2 mm (Figure 11.5). A new category of isolated tumor cells

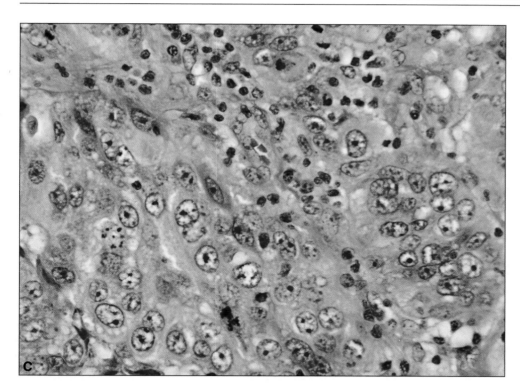

Figure 11.3. *(continued)*

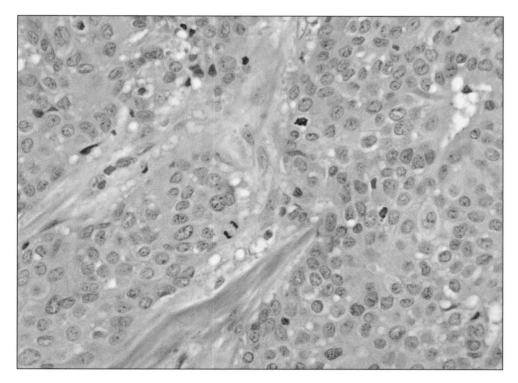

Figure 11.4. Mitotic figures in an invasive carcinoma, NST. Only dividing cells in which the mitotic figures can be readily identified in the division phase should be counted. Pyknotic nuclei should not be counted.

(ITC) was developed that corresponds to foci of tumor cells present on hematoxylin and eosin (H&E) and/or keratin immunohistochemistry, which measure less than 0.2 mm (Figure 11.6A–6C). The new staging category for these ITCs is N0$_{i+}$. The presence of extracapsular extension should be noted in lymph node

Figure 11.5. Micrometastatic carcinoma. This focus in the subcapsular sinus measures just short of 2 mm and thus qualifies as a micrometastasis.

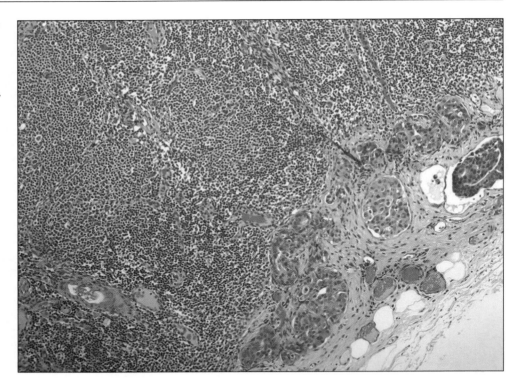

Figure 11.6. (A) Isolated tumor cells present in the subcapsular sinus of a lymph node. This small cluster of cells measures less than 0.2 mm and qualifies as isolated tumor cells (ITC) in the new staging system. (B,C) Keratin-positive cells in a sentinel lymph node (ITCs). In the first image, this focus of cells was only present on the slide stained with keratin. In the second image, a case of invasive lobular carcinoma was negative by H&E but rare keratin-positive cells are present on keratin immunohistochemistry.

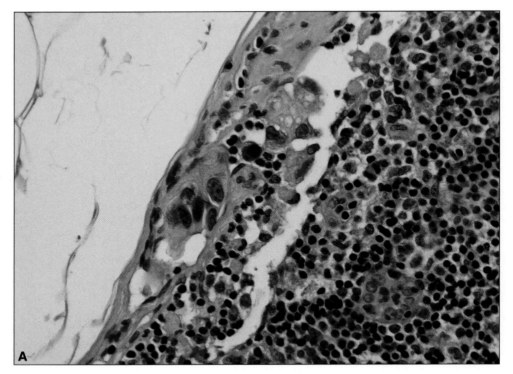

evaluations as this finding can be used to guide further therapy in certain situations (Figure 11.7).

Tumor size is an important prognostic factor and careful measurement of the invasive component is critical for proper staging. Gross measurements of

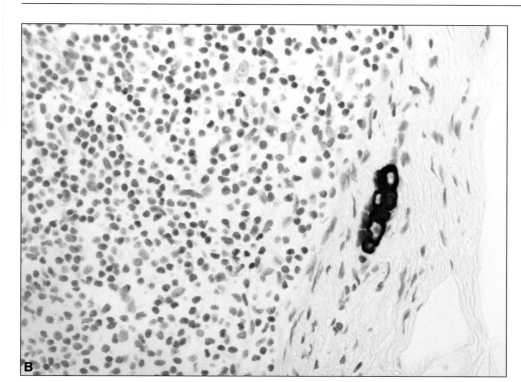

Figure 11.6. *(continued)*

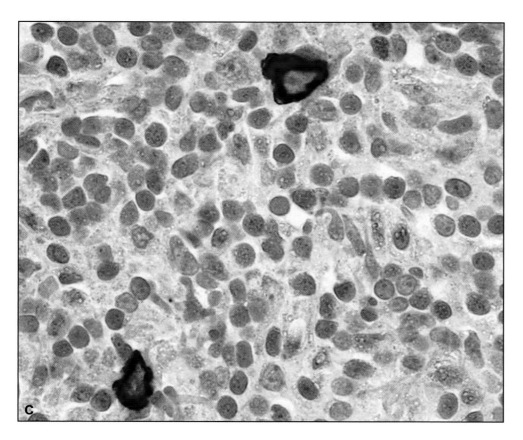

Figure 11.7. Extracapsular extension in a lymph node. Note the near-complete replacement of the node and the diffuse extension of carcinoma through the capsule into the surrounding fat.

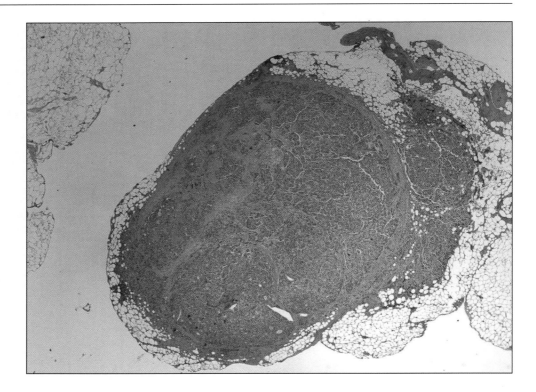

Figure 11.8. Estrogen receptor positivity in a grade I invasive mammary carcinoma, NST. Based on the Allred scoring system, this carcinoma overall had a positive score of 6.

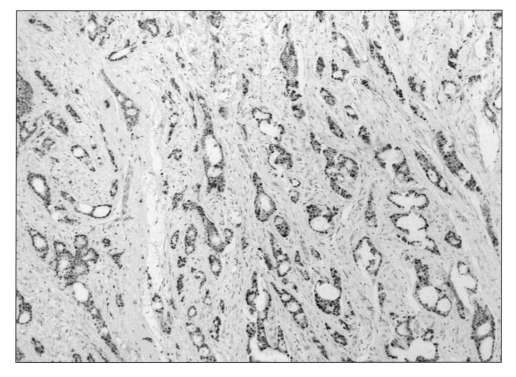

tumor size can be either under- or overestimated. Correlation with microscopic findings is critical as many carcinomas can have an admixture in ductal carcinoma in situ, which is not taken into consideration in tumor size for staging purposes. Also, many invasive carcinomas will have diffusely infiltrative

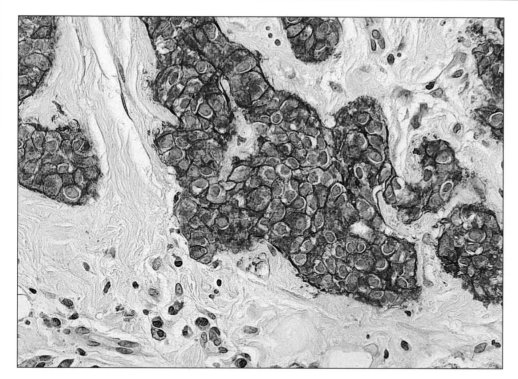

Figure 11.9.
Immunohistochemistry for c-erbB-2. Although it appears that there is a strong membrane staining in this case, it was scored 2+ because there was no circumferential, strong, linear staining of at least 30 percent of the tumor. The staining present here is somewhat weak and granular and not completely circumferential.

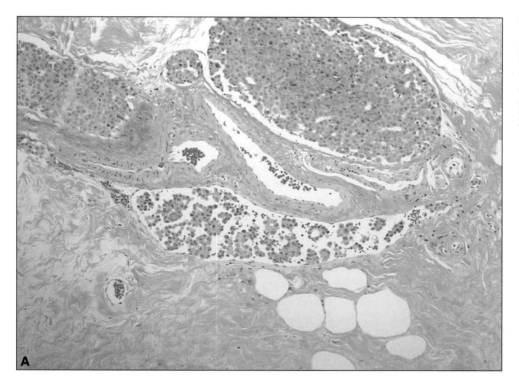

Figure 11.10.
(A,B) Angiolymphatic invasion in an invasive carcinoma, NST. Note the dilated vascular spaces plugged with markedly atypical epithelium.

borders and the microscopic measurement may be larger than the gross measurement.

Immunohistochemistry for estrogen/progesterone receptors (ER/PR) and c-erbB-2 should be performed on all invasive carcinomas based on a plethora of data

Figure 11.10. *(continued)*

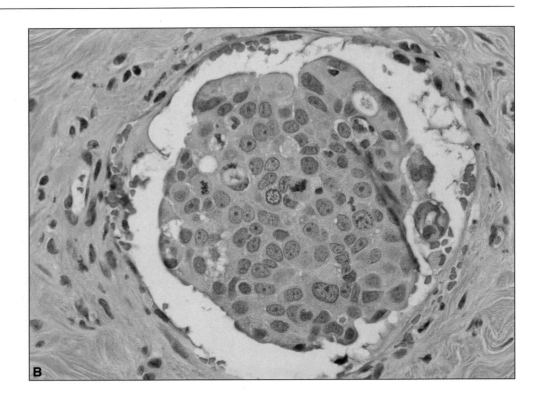

indicating the prognostic and predictive value of these markers. Unfortunately, there are a variety of antibodies for ER/PR in use and studies have shown variable results with different antibodies as well as with different fixation times. Currently, a universally accepted standard ER/PR antibody or a standard way of reporting positive or negative results is not available. We favor using the Allred score, based on strong clinical validation studies. In this method, the percentage of nuclei staining positive for estrogen receptor as well as the intensity of overall staining is combined for a score of 0, 2–8 (Figure 11.8). The importance of c-erbB-2 overexpression/amplification has received a great amount of attention in recent years, mainly due to the success of the monoclonal antibody drug treatment, herceptin, in patients who overexpress/amplify c-erbB-2. The importance of accurate results has led to recent changes in recommendations for c-erbB-2 testing by ASCO/CAP. Due to numerous studies, it is recommended that tissue submitted for c-erbB-2 immunohistochemistry be fixed in formalin for at least 6 h but not more than 48 h. In addition, although the scoring has not changed (0, 1–3+), the criteria have changed. For a 3+ overexpressing tumor, at least 30 percent of the cells should have strong, linear, and circumferential staining. In cases that do not fully meet this criterion (2+), FISH is recommended (Figure 11.9). In addition, the criteria for amplification of c-erbB-2 by FISH has changed with a ratio of 2.2 and above required for amplification and 1.8 and below being negative. The 1.8–2.2 range is now considered equivocal and additional testing should be performed.

Other markers, including proliferation markers, cell-cycle markers, and other oncogenes have been studied as prognostic and predictive markers in invasive carcinoma; however, based on a review by ASCO, there is insufficient data at this time to recommend these additional markers in the routine workup of invasive carcinomas of the breast. One exception to this is the multigene assay OncotypeDx,

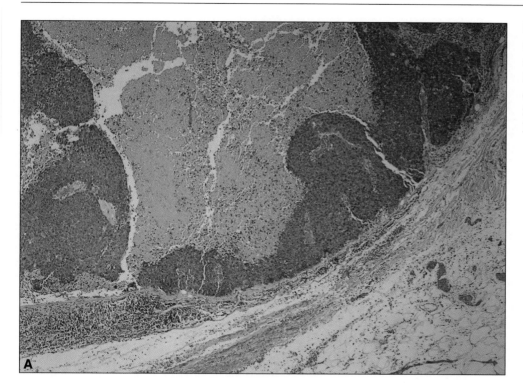

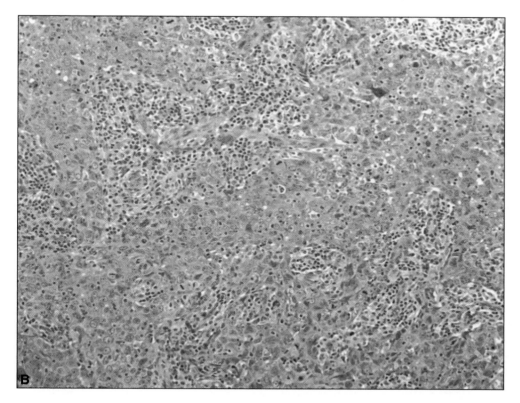

Figure 11.11.
(A,B) A triple-negative carcinoma in a patient with a BRCA1 mutation. The carcinoma has medullary features and was negative for ER/PR and c-erbB-2.

which in several studies has shown to aid in therapeutic decision-making regarding the use of chemotherapy in ER+, node-negative patients.

Finally, the presence of angiolymphatic invasion (ALI) in breast cancer has been shown to have prognostic significance (Figures 11.10A,B). Careful assessment of this finding is critical as many cancers will have "clefting" artifact, giving the appearance of carcinoma in vascular spaces.

INVASIVE CARCINOMA WITH BASAL PHENOTYPE

Recent studies using DNA microarray studies have helped define subsets of invasive mammary carcinoma, NST, including luminal types, which are generally ER/PR + and basal types, which are usually ER/PR− and negative for overexpression of c-erbB-2 (so-called triple-negative). In addition, the basal phenotype is associated with positive staining with myoepithelial type markers, including CK 5/6 and p63. These tumors are reported to have a worse prognosis when compared to luminal type tumors. Many of the tumors associated with BRCA1 mutations have this phenotype and can have a characteristic high-grade histology similar to medullary carcinomas (Figures 11.11A,B).

REFERENCES

Abdsaleh, S., F. Warnberg, et al. (2008). "Comparison of core needle biopsy and surgical specimens in malignant breast lesions regarding histological features and hormone receptor expression." *Histopathology* 52(6): 773–5.

Abner, A. L., L. Collins, et al. (1998). "Correlation of tumor size and axillary lymph node involvement with prognosis in patients with T1 breast carcinoma." *Cancer* 83(12): 2502–8.

Andrade, V. P. and H. Gobbi (2004). "Accuracy of typing and grading invasive mammary carcinomas on core needle biopsy compared with the excisional specimen." *Virchows Arch* 445(6): 597–602.

Barnes, D. M. and L. A. Newman (2007). "Pregnancy-associated breast cancer: a literature review." *Surg Clin North Am* 87(2): x, 417–30.

Bloom, H. J. and W. W. Richardson (1957). "Histological grading and prognosis in breast cancer: a study of 1409 cases of which 359 have been followed for 15 years." *Br J Cancer* 11(3): 359–77.

Carter, C. L., C. Allen, et al. (1989). "Relation of tumor size, lymph node status, and survival in 24,740 breast cancer cases." *Cancer* 63(1): 181–7.

Dalton, L. W., D. L. Page, et al. (1994). "Histologic grading of breast carcinoma. A reproducibility study." *Cancer* 73(11): 2765–70.

Diaz, L. K. and N. Sneige (2005). "Estrogen receptor analysis for breast cancer: current issues and keys to increasing testing accuracy." *Adv Anat Pathol* 12(1): 10–19.

Dunne, B. and J. J. Going (2001). "Scoring nuclear pleomorphism in breast cancer." *Histopathology* 39(3): 259–65.

Elston, C. W. and I. O. Ellis (1991). "Pathological prognostic factors in breast cancer. I. The value of histological grade in breast cancer: experience from a large study with long-term follow-up." *Histopathology* 19(5): 403–10.

Frierson, H. F., Jr., R. A. Wolber, et al. (1995). "Interobserver reproducibility of the Nottingham modification of the Bloom and Richardson histologic grading scheme for infiltrating ductal carcinoma." *Am J Clin Pathol* 103(2): 195–8.

Gajdos, C., P. I. Tartter, et al. (1999). "Lymphatic invasion, tumor size, and age are independent predictors of axillary lymph node metastases in women with T1 breast cancers." *Ann Surg* 230(5): 692–6.

Goldstein, N. S., M. Ferkowicz, et al. (2003). "Minimum formalin fixation time for consistent estrogen receptor immunohistochemical staining of invasive breast carcinoma." *Am J Clin Pathol* 120(1): 86–92.

Harris, L., H. Fritsche, et al. (2007). "American Society of Clinical Oncology 2007 update of recommendations for the use of tumor markers in breast cancer." *J Clin Oncol* 25(33): 5287–312.

Harvey, J. M., G. M. Clark, et al. (1999). "Estrogen receptor status by immunohistochemistry is superior to the ligand-binding assay for predicting response to adjuvant endocrine therapy in breast cancer." *J Clin Oncol* 17(5): 1474–81.

Hodi, Z., J. Chakrabarti, et al. (2007). "The reliability of assessment of oestrogen receptor expression on needle core biopsy specimens of invasive carcinomas of the breast." *J Clin Pathol* 60(3): 299–302.

Ito, M., T. Moriya, et al. (2007). "Significance of pathological evaluation for lymphatic vessel invasion in invasive breast cancer." *Breast Cancer* 14(4): 381–7.

Jacobs, T. W., K. P. Siziopikou, et al. (1998). "Do prognostic marker studies on core needle biopsy specimens of breast carcinoma accurately reflect the marker status of the tumor?" *Mod Pathol* 11(3): 259–64.

Kurosumi, M., K. Suemasu, et al. (2001). "Relationship between existence of lymphatic invasion in peritumoral breast tissue and presence of axillary lymph node metastasis in invasive ductal carcinoma of the breast." *Oncol Rep* 8(5): 1051–5.

Lee, A. H. and I. O. Ellis (2008). "The nottingham prognostic index for invasive carcinoma of the breast." *Pathol Oncol Res* 14(2): 113–15.

Lee, A. H., Z. Hodi, et al. (2008). "False-negative assessment of oestrogen receptor on needle core biopsy of invasive carcinoma of the breast." *J Clin Pathol* 61(2): 239–40.

Lee, A. K., R. A. DeLellis, et al. (1990). "Prognostic significance of peritumoral lymphatic and blood vessel invasion in node-negative carcinoma of the breast." *J Clin Oncol* 8(9): 1457–65.

Longacre, T. A., M. Ennis, et al. (2006). "Interobserver agreement and reproducibility in classification of invasive breast carcinoma: an NCI breast cancer family registry study." *Mod Pathol* 19(2): 195–207.

Mann, G. B., V. D. Fahey, et al. (2005). "Reliance on hormone receptor assays of surgical specimens may compromise outcome in patients with breast cancer." *J Clin Oncol* 23(22): 5148–54.

Monticciolo, D. L. (2005). "Histologic grading at breast core needle biopsy: comparison with results from the excised breast specimen." *Breast J* 11(1): 9–14.

Paik, S., S. Shak, et al. (2004). "A multigene assay to predict recurrence of tamoxifen-treated, node-negative breast cancer." *N Engl J Med* 351(27): 2817–26.

Paik, S., G. Tang, et al. (2006). "Gene expression and benefit of chemotherapy in women with node-negative, estrogen receptor-positive breast cancer." *J Clin Oncol* 24(23): 3726–34.

Park, S. Y., K. S. Kim, et al. (2008). "The accuracy of preoperative core biopsy in determining histologic grade, hormone receptors, and human epidermal growth factor receptor 2 status in invasive breast cancer." *Am J Surg*.

Pinder, S. E., I. O. Ellis, et al. (1994). "Pathological prognostic factors in breast cancer. III. Vascular invasion: relationship with recurrence and survival in a large study with long-term follow-up." *Histopathology* 24(1): 41–7.

Pinder, S. E., S. Murray, et al. (1998). "The importance of the histologic grade of invasive breast carcinoma and response to chemotherapy." *Cancer* 83(8): 1529–39.

Rakha, E. A. and I. O. Ellis (2007). "An overview of assessment of prognostic and predictive factors in breast cancer needle core biopsy specimens." *J Clin Pathol* 60(12): 1300–6.

Rakha, E. A., M. E. El-Sayed, et al. (2008). "Prognostic significance of Nottingham histologic grade in invasive breast carcinoma." *J Clin Oncol* 26(19): 3153–8.

Rakha, E. A., J. S. Reis-Filho, et al. (2008). "Basal-like breast cancer: a critical review." *J Clin Oncol* 26(15): 2568–81.

Rhodes, A., B. Jasani, et al. (2001). "Study of interlaboratory reliability and reproducibility of estrogen and progesterone receptor assays in Europe. Documentation of poor reliability and identification of insufficient microwave antigen retrieval time as a major contributory element of unreliable assays." *Am J Clin Pathol* 115(1): 44–58.

Say, C. C. and W. L. Donegan (1974). "Invasive carcinoma of the breast: prognostic significance of tumor size and involved axillary lymph nodes." *Cancer* 34(2): 468–71.

Singletary, S. E., C. Allred, et al. (2002). "Revision of the American Joint Committee on Cancer staging system for breast cancer." *J Clin Oncol* 20(17): 3628–36.

Sloane, J. P., I. Amendoeira, et al. (1999). "Consistency achieved by 23 European pathologists from 12 countries in diagnosing breast disease and reporting prognostic features of carcinomas. European Commission Working Group on Breast Screening Pathology." *Virchows Arch* 434(1): 3–10.

Sorlie, T., C. M. Perou, et al. (2001). "Gene expression patterns of breast carcinomas distinguish tumor subclasses with clinical implications." *Proc Natl Acad Sci USA* 98(19): 10869–74.

Striebel, J. M., R. Bhargava, et al. (2008). "The equivocally amplified HER2 FISH result on breast core biopsy: indications for further sampling do affect patient management." *Am J Clin Pathol* 129(3): 383–90.

Tsuda, H., F. Akiyama, et al. (1999). "Monitoring of interobserver agreement in nuclear atypia scoring of node-negative breast carcinomas judged at individual collaborating hospitals in the National Surgical Adjuvant Study of Breast Cancer (NSAS-BC) protocol." *Jpn J Clin Oncol* 29(9): 413–20.

van Diest, P. J., J. P. Baak, et al. (1992). "Reproducibility of mitosis counting in 2,469 breast cancer specimens: results from the Multicenter Morphometric Mammary Carcinoma Project." *Hum Pathol* 23(6): 603–7.

Wolff, A. C., M. E. Hammond, et al. (2007). "American Society of Clinical Oncology/College of American Pathologists guideline recommendations for human epidermal growth factor receptor 2 testing in breast cancer." *J Clin Oncol* 25(1): 118–45.

12 METAPLASTIC CARCINOMA AND SARCOMA

Thomas J. Lawton, MD

Metaplastic Carcinoma	199
Spindle Cell Carcinoma	199
Squamous Cell Carcinoma	203
Metaplastic Carcinoma with Osteochondroid	
Differentiation	203
Sarcoma	205

METAPLASTIC CARCINOMA

Metaplastic carcinomas are a diverse group of invasive carcinomas with varied histologies including spindle cell, squamous cell, and/or heterologous elements such as osteoid or chondroid differentiation. Often, the tumors are composed of a component of invasive mammary carcinoma, no special type (NST), which is identified in association with the metaplastic elements; however, sometimes this finding can be very focal or absent and the differential diagnosis includes other entities such as primary sarcoma of the breast, a rare disease. The clinical and radiographic presentation as well as the age at diagnosis does not differ significantly from patients with invasive mammary carcinoma, NST.

Spindle Cell Carcinoma

Spindle cell carcinomas have varied histology, some showing an association of the spindle cell component with an area of invasive mammary carcinoma, NST, ductal carcinoma in situ (DCIS), or squamous differentiation admixed with the spindled component, and others where the lesion is entirely spindled and the differential includes other spindled neoplasms of the breast (monophasic). One type of monophasic spindle cell carcinoma has a very low-grade appearance akin to fibromatosis (Figures 12.1A–C). Immunohistochemistry with a battery of keratin markers, including broad-spectrum cytokeratin and in particular high-molecular-weight cytokeratin, can aid in this distinction as fibromatosis is negative for keratins (Figure 12.1D); additional staining with β-catenin, positive in approximately 80 percent of cases of fibromatosis, may assist in excluding this diagnosis if the

Figure 12.1. (A) Low-grade fibromatosis-like spindle cell carcinoma. Note the infiltrative nature of the lesion and the low-grade cytology of the spindle cells. (B,C) Low-grade fibromatosis-like spindle cell carcinoma with fascicles of spindles with relatively bland nuclei without significant pleomorphism. (D) Diffuse keratin positivity in low-grade fibromatosis-like spindle cell carcinoma.

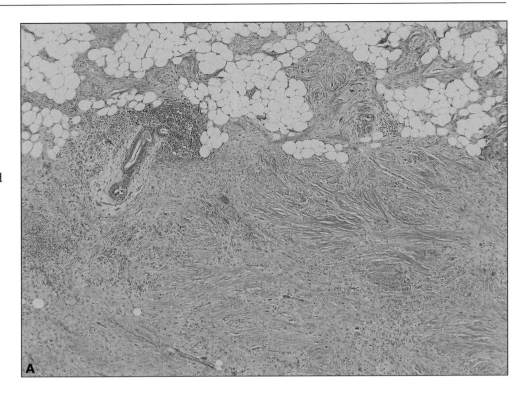

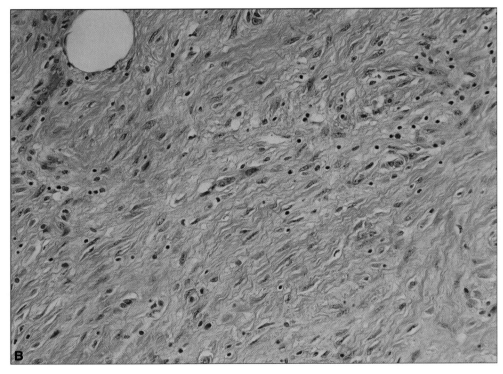

result shows strong nuclear positivity. Although bland in appearance, these lesions can recur and distant metastases have been reported; thus, it is recommended these patients undergo excision with adequate margins and sentinel lymph node biopsy. These tumors are usually triple-negative.

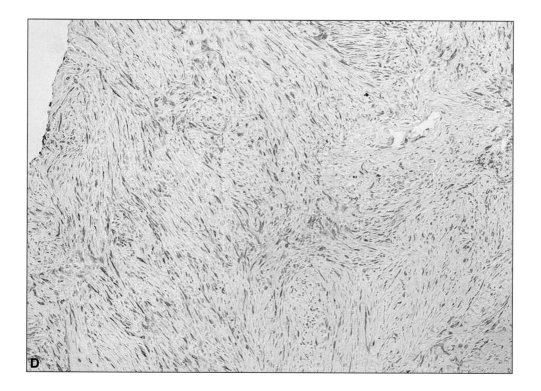

Figure 12.1. *(continued)*

Other spindle cell carcinomas can have higher grade cytology, with plump, pleomorphic cells that blend in with an area of usual invasive mammary carcinoma, NST, DCIS, or areas of squamous differentiation (Figure 12.2). When an epithelial component is readily identified, the diagnosis is usually straightforward;

Figure 12.2. High-grade
biphasic spindle cell
carcinoma. A high-grade
spindled cell area blends
imperceptively with a high-
grade epithelial component of
carcinoma.

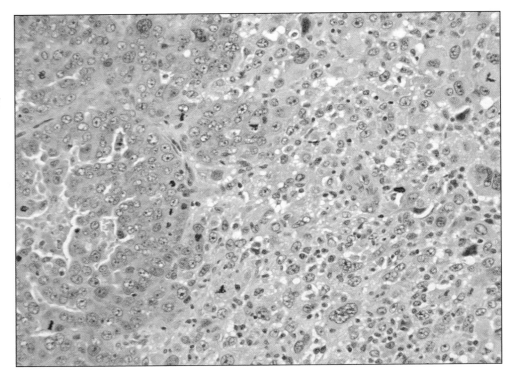

Figure 12.3. (A,B) Spindle
cell carcinoma, monophasic.
A pleomorphic population of
spindle cells is present
adjacent to a benign duct.
Keratin immunostain reveals
the epithelial nature of the
process and confirms the
diagnosis of spindle cell
carcinoma.

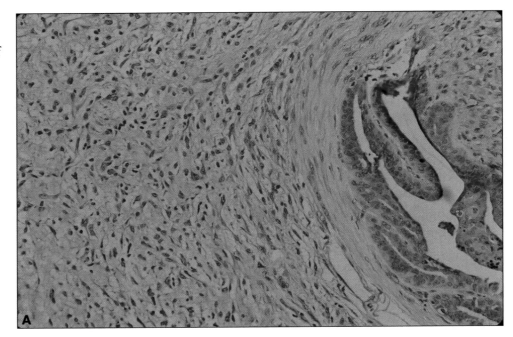

however, extensive sampling of the lesion should be performed as these areas of
usual invasive mammary carcinoma, NST, or DCIS can be focal. In cases of pure
spindle cell carcinoma, the differential includes a primary sarcoma of the breast
and keratin immunohistochemistry, as reviewed for low-grade fibromatosis-like
carcinoma, is helpful (Figures 12.3A,B). Surgical excision with clear margins and
sentinel lymph node biopsy is recommended.

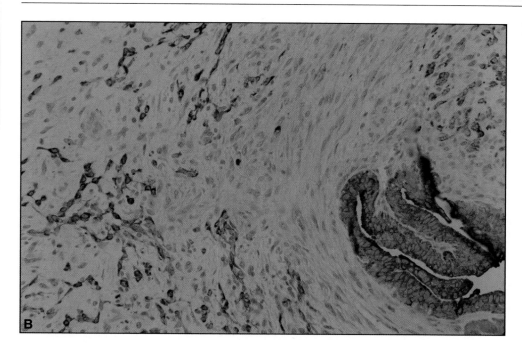

Figure 12.3. *(continued)*

Spindle cell carcinomas of the breast are usually triple-negative (ER-/PR- and c-erbB-2-negative). There is some suggestion of myoepithelial differentiation and a basal phenotype based on some immunohistochemical studies.

Squamous Cell Carcinoma

Squamous cell carcinoma is a type of metaplastic carcinoma that is similar in histology to squamous cell carcinomas in extramammary sites. Grossly, these lesions frequently appear cystic. The sections will show a tumor composed of nests of malignant squamous epithelium often blending in with a spindle-cell component (Figure 12.4). In the latter circumstance, keratin immunohistochemistry can aid in confirming the epithelial nature of the associated spindle cells. Pure squamous cell carcinomas of the breast are uncommon and thus data on follow-up is limited although the existing data suggest a prognosis not unlike usual invasive mammary carcinoma, NST, of similar stage. Treatment should consist of surgical excision with adequate margins and sentinel lymph node biopsy.

Metaplastic Carcinoma with Osteochondroid Differentiation

These tumors, often called matrix-producing carcinomas, are composed usually of a high-grade carcinoma blending with an osseous or cartilaginous matrix (Figures 12.5A,B). Matrix-producing carcinoma with chondroid matrix frequently has the low-power appearance of being multinodular and relatively circumscribed (Figure 12.6A). Toward the periphery, high-grade epithelioid cells are present in nests and

Figure 12.4. Squamous cell carcinoma. Nests of malignant squamous epithelium are present infiltrating the stroma. Toward the lower right, the neoplasm takes on a more spindled cell appearance.

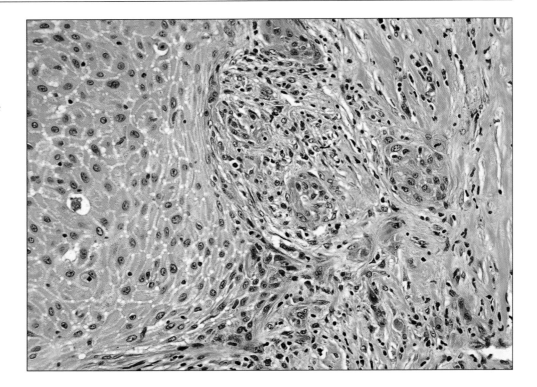

Figure 12.5. Metaplastic carcinoma with osteo–chondroid differentiation. The high-grade invasive carcinoma blends with areas of osseous differentiation (A) and chondroid differentiation (B).

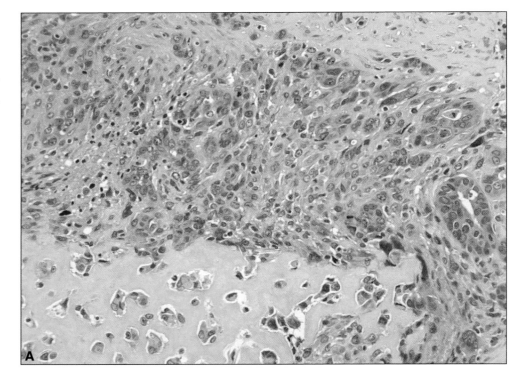

trabeculae within the chondroid matrix. These cells stain positively for cytokeratins. The matrix stains positively for S-100. As with other metaplastic carcinomas, treatment includes surgical excision with adequate margins and sentinel lymph node biopsy.

Figure 12.5. *(continued)*

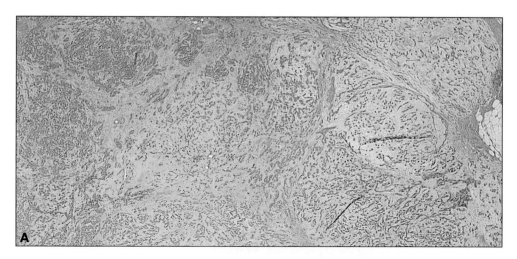

Figure 12.6.
(A,B) Matrix-producing carcinoma. At low power, the neoplasm has a multinodular appearance with a more central area of chondroid matrix. The cells at high power are high grade with pleomorphic nuclei and mitotic activity growing in small nests and trabeculae.

SARCOMA

Primary sarcomas of the breast are extremely rare, accounting for less than 0.1 percent of all malignancies in the breast. Angiosarcoma is the most common of these and the rest, which show identical histology to their counterparts in an extramammary location, will not be discussed in this chapter due to their rarity. When confronted with a probable primary sarcoma of the breast, consultation with an expert in bone and soft tissue pathology is recommended.

Figure 12.6. *(continued)*

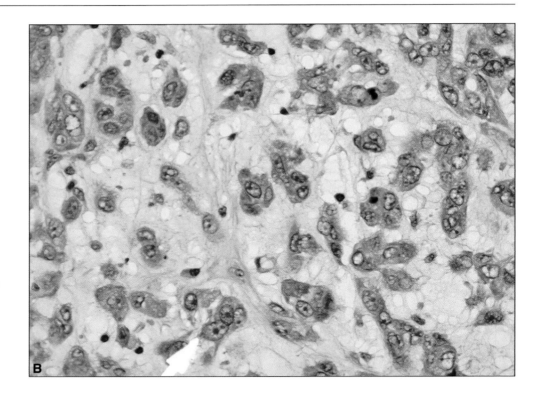

Figure 12.7. (A–C) Low-grade angiosarcoma. A diffusely infiltrative process composed of anastamosing open vascular channels with minimal endothelial cell atypia, no solid growth, and no endothelial tufting or papillary growth.

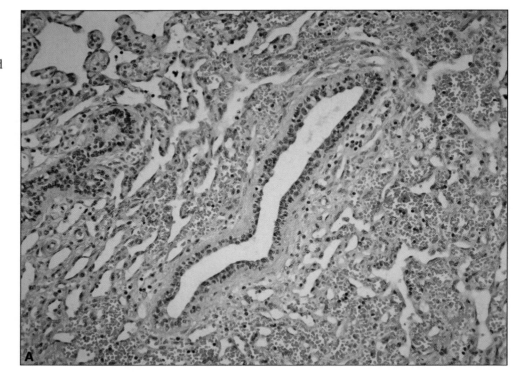

Primary angiosarcoma is the most common type and generally occurs in patients at a younger age than secondary angiosarcomas, which are secondary malignancies following radiotherapy for breast carcinoma. These tumors can be parenchymal but frequently are located in the dermis where they can present as a

Figure 12.7. *(continued)*

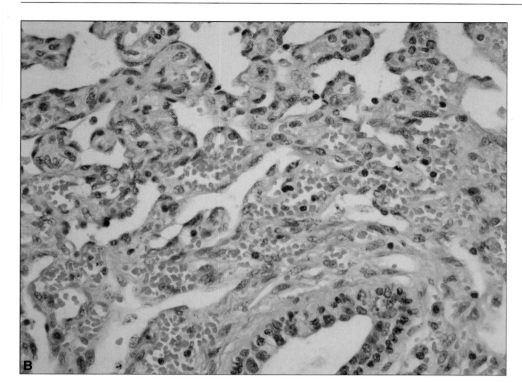

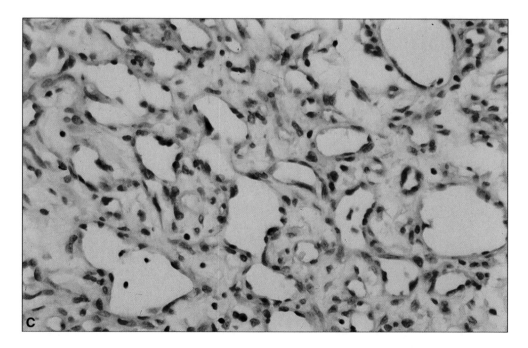

bluish-purplish discoloration on the skin. Lastly, Stewart-Treves syndrome refers to angiosarcomas arising secondary to lymphedema in the arm. The imaging findings are nonspecific and often show a mass lesion but may be negative.

Histologically, angiosarcomas are a diverse set of tumors, which are classically divided into three grades (low, intermediate, and high). Angiosarcomas have permeative growth patterns, surrounding and invading adjacent lobules. Low-grade

Figure 12.8.
(A,B) Intermediate-grade
angiosarcoma. The tumor is
similar to that in Figure 12.7
but there are focal areas of
solid growth and scattered
mitotic activity within the
mildly pleomorphic
endothelial cells.

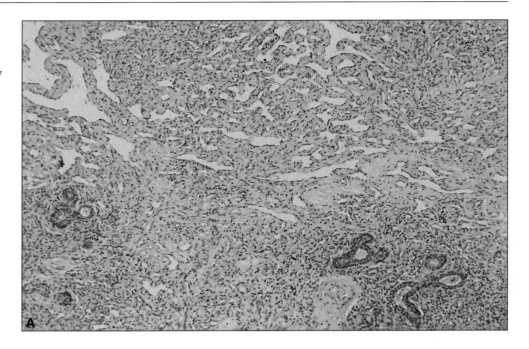

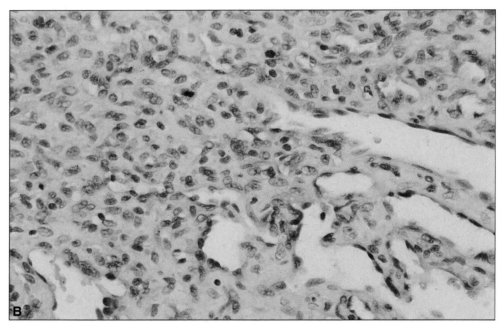

angiosarcomas are characterized by an anastamosing pattern of open vascular channels with only mild endothelial atypia and rare to absent mitotic figures. No endothelial cell tufting or papillary growth is seen (Figures 12.7A–C). Intermediate-grade angiosarcomas have similar appearances to low-grade angiosarcomas although there can be papillary growth, focal solid areas, and some mitotic activity within the endothelial cells (Figures 12.8A,B). High-grade angiosarcomas are characterized by marked endothelial cell atypia, mitotic activity, solid areas of growth, necrosis, and "blood" lakes (Figures 12.9A–C).

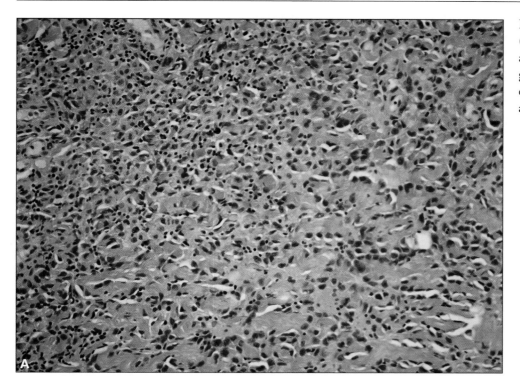

Figure 12.9. (A–C) High-grade angiosarcoma. Extensive solid growth pattern with endothelial tufting, marked atypia, and "blood lakes."

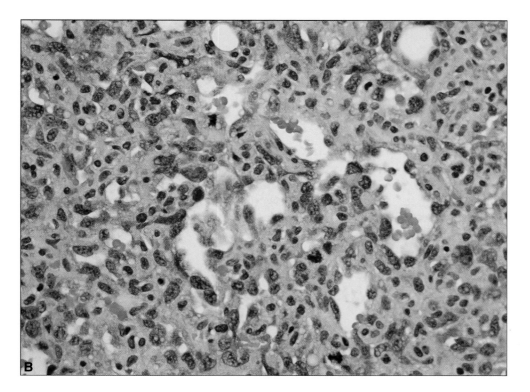

The differential on the low-grade end of the spectrum is with atypical hemangiomas/atypical vascular lesions, pseudoangiomatous stromal hyperplasia (PASH), and cellular angiolipoma. Atypical hemangiomas generally are small lesions that are usually circumscribed and lack the invasive border of angiosarcoma. Atypical

Figure 12.9. *(continued)*

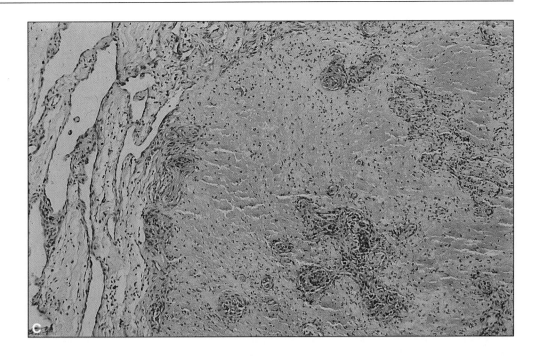

vascular lesions are uncommon lesions following radiation therapy and are most likely confused with secondary angiosarcoma. Although this differential can be hard, generally these lesions are lobulated or circumscribed, and lack infiltrative borders. PASH is a lesion composed of myofibroblastic cells lining slit-like spaces, which can be confused with low-grade angiosarcoma; however, immunohistochemistry can aid in this distinction as PASH is not a vascular neoplasm. On the high-grade end of the spectrum, angiosarcoma can be confused with a high- grade infiltrating carcinoma or other sarcoma. Keratin immunohistochemistry should be negative (but not always) in angiosarcomas and vascular markers should be positive.

The treatment of angiosarcoma includes surgical excision with adequate margins. Since these tumors can be diffusely infiltrative and large, mastectomy is often the choice of surgical procedure. As in other sarcomas, axillary nodal evaluation is not recommended as these tumors rarely involve the axillary nodes. Postoperative chemotherapy and radiation therapy are controversial. Prognosis is dependent on tumor grade and size.

REFERENCES

Adem, C., C. Reynolds, et al. (2002). "Wide spectrum screening keratin as a marker of metaplastic spindle cell carcinoma of the breast: an immunohistochemical study of 24 patients." *Histopathology* 40(6): 556–62.

Adem, C., C. Reynolds, et al. (2004). "Primary breast sarcoma: clinicopathologic series from the Mayo Clinic and review of the literature." *Br J Cancer* 91(2): 237–41.

Carter, M. R., J. L. Hornick, et al. (2006). "Spindle cell (sarcomatoid) carcinoma of the breast: a clinicopathologic and immunohistochemical analysis of 29 cases." *Am J Surg Pathol* 30(3): 300–9.

Chhieng, C., M. Cranor, et al. (1998). "Metaplastic carcinoma of the breast with osteocartilaginous heterologous elements." *Am J Surg Pathol* 22(2): 188–94.

Christensen, L., T. Schiodt, et al. (1988). "Sarcomas of the breast: a clinico-pathological study of 67 patients with long term follow-up." *Eur J Surg Oncol* 14(3): 241–7.

Dunne, B., A. H. Lee, et al. (2003). "An immunohistochemical study of metaplastic spindle cell carcinoma, phyllodes tumor and fibromatosis of the breast." *Hum Pathol* 34(10): 1009–15.

Gobbi, H., J. F. Simpson, et al. (1999). "Metaplastic breast tumors with a dominant fibromatosis-like phenotype have a high risk of local recurrence." *Cancer* 85(10): 2170–82.

Hennessy, B. T., S. Giordano, et al. (2006). "Biphasic metaplastic sarcomatoid carcinoma of the breast." *Ann Oncol* 17(4): 605–13.

Kiluk, J. V. and K. A. Yeh (2005). "Primary angiosarcoma of the breast." *Breast J* 11(6): 517–18.

Koker, M. M. and C. G. Kleer (2004). "p63 expression in breast cancer: a highly sensitive and specific marker of metaplastic carcinoma." *Am J Surg Pathol* 28(11): 1506–12.

Kurian, K. M. and A. Al-Nafussi (2002). "Sarcomatoid/metaplastic carcinoma of the breast: a clinicopathological study of 12 cases." *Histopathology* 40(1): 58–64.

Kuroda, N., N. Fujishima, et al. (2008). "Basal-like carcinoma of the breast: further evidence of the possibility that most metaplastic carcinomas may be actually basal-like carcinomas." *Med Mol Morphol* 41(2): 117–20.

Leibl, S., M. Gogg-Kammerer, et al. (2005). "Metaplastic breast carcinomas: are they of myoepithelial differentiation? Immunohistochemical profile of the sarcomatoid subtype using novel myoepithelial markers." *Am J Surg Pathol* 29(3): 347–53.

Luini, A., G. Gatti, et al. (2007). "Angiosarcoma of the breast: the experience of the European Institute of Oncology and a review of the literature." *Breast Cancer Res Treat* 105(1): 81–5.

Merino, M. J., D. Carter, et al. (1983). "Angiosarcoma of the breast." *Am J Surg Pathol* 7(1): 53–60.

Naka, N., M. Ohsawa, et al. (1996). "Prognostic factors in angiosarcoma: a multivariate analysis of 55 cases." *J Surg Oncol* 61(3): 170–6.

Oberman, H. A. (1987). "Metaplastic carcinoma of the breast. A clinicopathologic study of 29 patients." *Am J Surg Pathol* 11(12): 918–29.

Ostrowski, J. L., K. Horgan, et al. (1998). "Monophasic sarcomatoid carcinoma of the breast." *Histopathology* 32(2): 184–6.

Pitts, W. C., V. A. Rojas, et al. (1991). "Carcinomas with metaplasia and sarcomas of the breast." *Am J Clin Pathol* 95(5): 623–32.

Pollard, S. G., P. V. Marks, et al. (1990). "Breast sarcoma. A clinicopathologic review of 25 cases." *Cancer* 66(5): 941–4.

Rakha, E. A., T. C. Putti, et al. (2006). "Morphological and immunophenotypic analysis of breast carcinomas with basal and myoepithelial differentiation." *J Pathol* 208(4): 495–506.

Rosen, P. P., M. Kimmel, et al. (1988). "Mammary angiosarcoma. The prognostic significance of tumor differentiation." *Cancer* 62(10): 2145–51.

Sneige, N., H. Yaziji, et al. (2001). "Low-grade (fibromatosis-like) spindle cell carcinoma of the breast." *Am J Surg Pathol* 25(8): 1009–16.

Tse, G. M., P. H. Tan, et al. (2006). "Metaplastic carcinoma of the breast: a clinicopathological review." *J Clin Pathol* 59(10): 1079–83.

Vorburger, S. A., Y. Xing, et al. (2005). "Angiosarcoma of the breast." *Cancer* 104(12): 2682–8.

Wargotz, E. S., P. H. Deos, et al. (1989). "Metaplastic carcinomas of the breast. II. Spindle cell carcinoma." *Hum Pathol* 20(8): 732–40.

Wargotz, E. S. and H. J. Norris (1989). "Metaplastic carcinomas of the breast. I. Matrix-producing carcinoma." *Hum Pathol* 20(7): 628–35.

Wargotz, E. S. and H. J. Norris (1989). "Metaplastic carcinomas of the breast. III. Carcinosarcoma." *Cancer* 64(7): 1490–9.

Wargotz, E. S. and H. J. Norris (1990). "Metaplastic carcinomas of the breast. IV. Squamous cell carcinoma of ductal origin." *Cancer* 65(2): 272–6.

13 CYTOLOGY OF THE BREAST

Elena Brachtel, MD

Clinical Indications and Limitations	213
Terminology/Reporting	214
Sample Preparation	214
Fibroepithelial Lesions	216
Papillary Lesions	219
Proliferative Epithelial Lesions, Including those with "Atypia"	219
Carcinoma	225
Metaplastic, Mesenchymal, and Spindle Cell Lesions	230
Newer Technologies	230
Hormone Receptor and HER-2 Studies in Breast Cancer Diagnostics	230
Ductal Lavage Cytology and Nipple Fluid Analysis	234
Use of Imprint Cytology (Touch Prep) in Intraoperative Consultation: Margin Assessment and Sentinel Node Evaluation	234

CLINICAL INDICATIONS AND LIMITATIONS

The use of breast cytology as a primary diagnostic tool for breast lesions seems to be declining with core biopsies replacing fine needle aspirations of the breast for primary tissue diagnosis. However, fine needle aspiration biopsies of breast lesions have high utility for diagnosis and triage, and may be the method of choice in situations when a core biopsy does not seem to be indicated. Imprint cytology can play an important role in rapid diagnosis of surgical breast specimens. Also, the favorable cost-effectiveness of cytologic sampling is to be taken into account. There are many reasons why the skill to interpret breast cytology must not be neglected.

- High sensitivity and specificity when interpreted by skilled cytologists
- Tissue diagnosis for palpable breast lesions (very low false-negative rate when used as part of triple test)

- Triage and immediate confirmation of malignancy in clinically suspicious breast lesions
- Imprint cytology on sentinel lymph nodes and surgical margins
- Cytologic sampling of axillary lymph nodes
- Metastatic lesions and recurrences
- Risk assessment in patients at high risk for breast cancer

TERMINOLOGY/REPORTING

The first step is to establish if the sample is of satisfactory quality and cellularity to allow a resolution of the clinical problem. A quality indicator in the report is useful to confirm that the sample is satisfactory for evaluation, or to give reasons that limit the evaluation (e.g., low cellularity, scant epithelial cells, or obscuring inflammation).

A probabilistic approach in reporting of breast cytology samples allows well-defined diagnostic categories for most specimens:

- Nondiagnostic
- Benign or no malignant cells identified (specific diagnosis more reliable)
- Atypical (specimen that is probably benign but requires confirmation)
- Suspicious (specimen that is probably malignant but there are too few cells, poorly preserved, or other limiting factors).
- Positive for malignant cells

The necessity to correlate cytologic findings with clinical and radiographic features (triple test) cannot be overemphasized. Radiologic reports follow BIRADS categories 0 to 5, which can be correlated with the cytology result. Most false-negative breast cytology tests were found to be due to inadequate sampling, with consequences that may be prevented by careful correlation with clinical findings.

Normal breast tissue produces scant aspirates but several groups of ductal epithelial cells should be represented. In benign breast parenchyma or lesions, ductal epithelial cells are accompanied by myoepithelial cells, often also referred to as bipolar cells or naked nuclei (Figures 13.1 and 13.2).

SAMPLE PREPARATION

Breast cytology samples can be processed as direct smears or thin-layer preparation. Direct smears are ethanol-fixed and stained with Papanicolaou, hematoxylin, and eosin, or air-dried and Giemsa-stained (the latter providing less nuclear detail).

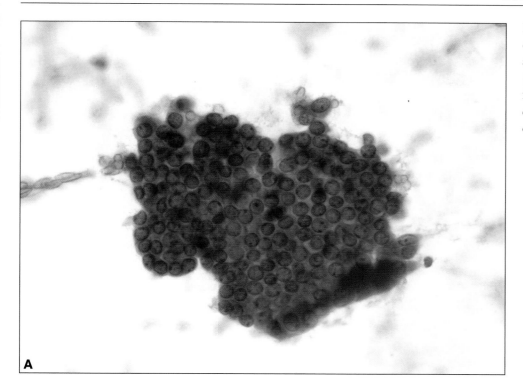

Figure 13.1. (A,B) Benign ductal epithelial cells with associated myoepithelial cells (same group with a different focus shows the myoepithelial cells overlying the epithelial cells).

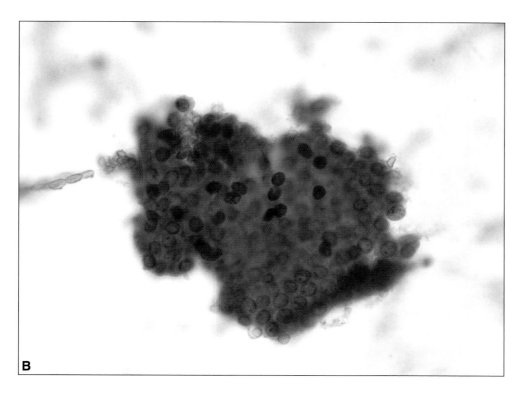

Liquid-based cytology is based on filtration or sedimentation methods. Direct smears and liquid-based cytology have inherent advantages and disadvantages, but are considered of comparable diagnostic value. The method of choice for a laboratory depends on usual practice, preference, and resources. When viewing

Figure 13.2. Benign lobule with myoepithelial cells in the background.

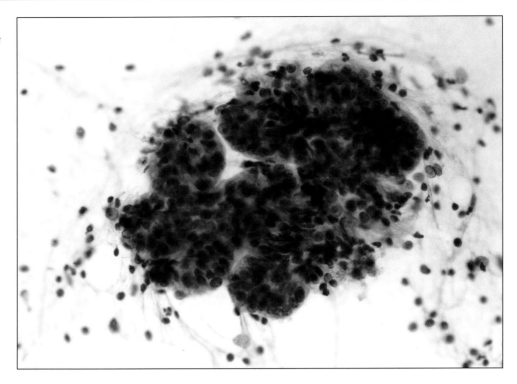

thin-layer preparations, certain morphological alterations should be taken into account (Figures 13.3–4):

- Loss of architecture
- Fragmentation and three-dimensional appearance of cell groups
- "Clean" background with apparent lack of myoepithelial cells

FIBROEPITHELIAL LESIONS

A fibroepithelial lesion is composed of an epithelial and a stromal component, and most frequently represents a fibroadenoma (Figures 13.5–7). Typical (but not necessarily specific) cytologic features of fibroadenoma include the following:

- Large groups of epithelial cells, often in "staghorn" or "animal" shapes
- Myoepithelial cells associated with epithelial groups and in the background
- Stromal fragments

The differential diagnosis of a benign fibroepithelial lesion includes hamartoma, pseudoangiomatous stromal hyperplasia (PASH), or fibrocystic changes; the cytomorphological features may be indistinguishable.

There are diagnostic pitfalls in the context of fibroadenomas that the cytologist needs to be aware of. The remarkable hypercellularity of the smear could

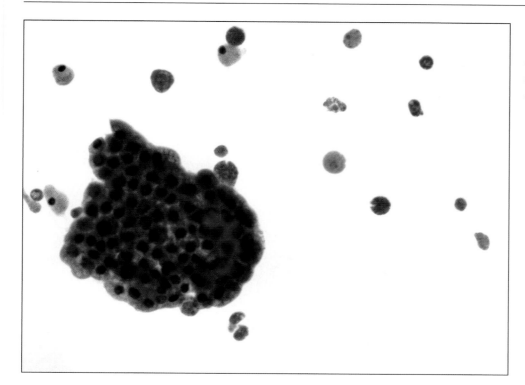

Figure 13.3. ThinPrep® of fluid from a benign breast cyst – ductal cells with apocrine metaplasia and foam cells.

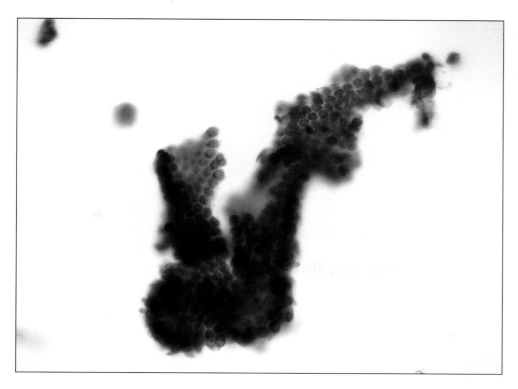

Figure 13.4. SurePath® of a breast mass – three-dimensional appearance of the cellular groups.

lead to the interpretation of a fibroadenoma on cytology as "malignant": bland epithelial components and the background of myoepithelial cells will help distinguish this from carcinoma. Occasional atypical or multinucleated stromal cells can be seen in fibroadenomas (Figure 13.8). Hypercellular stromal fragments

Figure 13.5. Fibroadenoma. The cellular smear shows "animal-shaped" large sheets of cohesive ductal epithelial cells with a sprinkling of myoepithelial cells in the background and few stromal fragments.

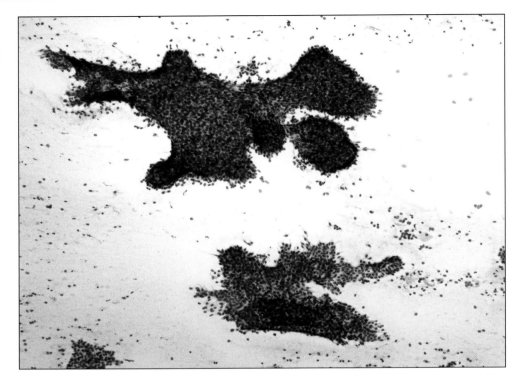

Figure 13.6. Fibroadenoma. Ductal epithelium is attached to a stromal fragment.

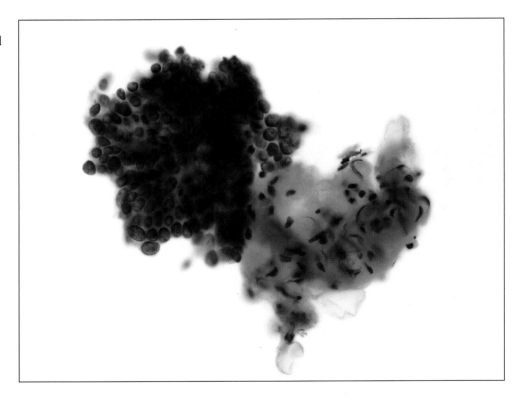

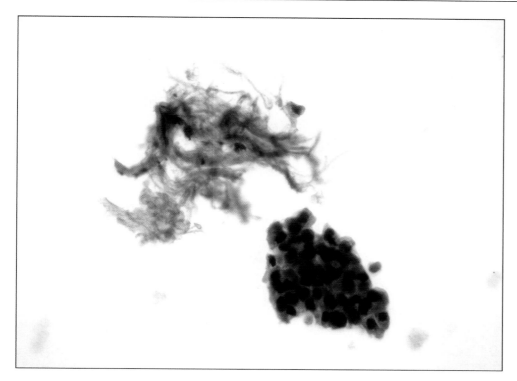

Figure 13.7. The thin-layer preparation (ThinPrep®) essentially shows similar features but the characteristic large epithelial sheets of fibroadenoma are often present in smaller fragments and the background lacks myoepithelial cells.

with atypical stromal cells in a growing mass may raise the possibility of a phyllodes tumor (Figure 13.9). In those cases, atypical features should be mentioned.

PAPILLARY LESIONS

Papillary fragments appear as finger-like, rounded cell clusters on cytology. Fibrovascular cores, the hallmark of papillary lesions, are obvious when seen on histologic section, but are often not appreciated on cytology (Figures 13.10–12).

Papillary lesions can range from benign intraductal papilloma that typically present with bloody nipple discharge, to invasive papillary carcinoma and micropapillary carcinoma (Figure 13.13). Carcinoma may be associated with more cellular samples, nuclear atypia, and complex papillary structures.

Not always do papillary fragments on cytology correspond to papillary lesions on excision. The underlying pathology may indeed represent a benign intraductal papilloma, but fibrocystic changes, fibroadenoma, or other benign lesions often occur. A true papilloma on excision may not show "papillary" fragments on cytology.

PROLIFERATIVE EPITHELIAL LESIONS, INCLUDING THOSE WITH "ATYPIA"

Proliferative breast lesions are considered "without atypia" if small, uniform epithelial cells with round or ovoid nuclei, smooth nuclear contours, even chromatin

Figure 13.8. Fibroepithelial lesion with atypical stromal cells. Benign-appearing epithelial groups were in the background (A). A high-power view shows large, atypical mesenchymal-type cells (B).

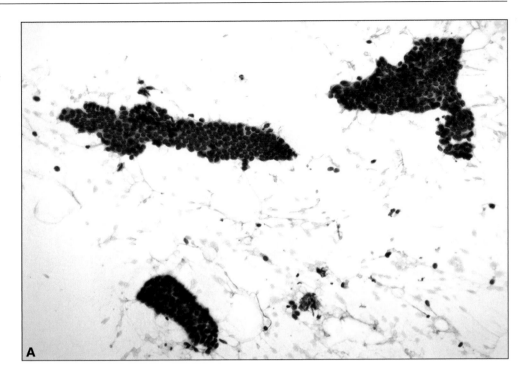

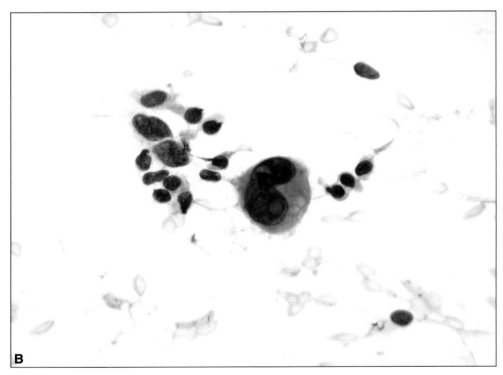

distribution, and variable nuclear-to-cytoplasmic ratios are present in sheets of not more than two-cell layers and accompanied by myoepithelial cells. Atypical features include nuclear enlargement and variability, granular chromatin texture, and nucleoli and nuclear crowding (Figures 13.14–16). However, the "atypical" category is

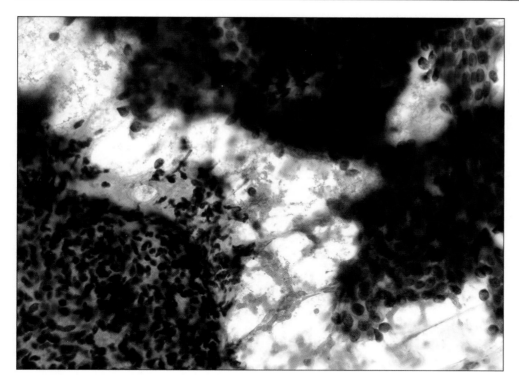

Figure 13.9. Suspicious for phyllodes tumor. Hypercellular stromal fragment and hyperplastic ductal epithelium.

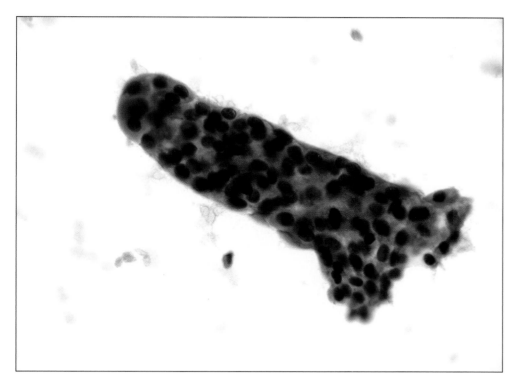

Figure 13.10. Intraductal Papilloma. The finger-like papillary fragment shows ductal epithelial cells with cohesive, small, oval nuclei and occasional myoepithelial cells.

problematic and has been shown to have low interobserver agreement even among experienced cytopathologists.

Ductal proliferations may be difficult to diagnose even on surgical material, where ancillary tests such as immunohistochemical stains are often used. In cytology,

Figure 13.11. Intraductal papilloma. The ThinPrep® shows poorly preserved, rounded epithelial groups, and a foamy histiocyte.

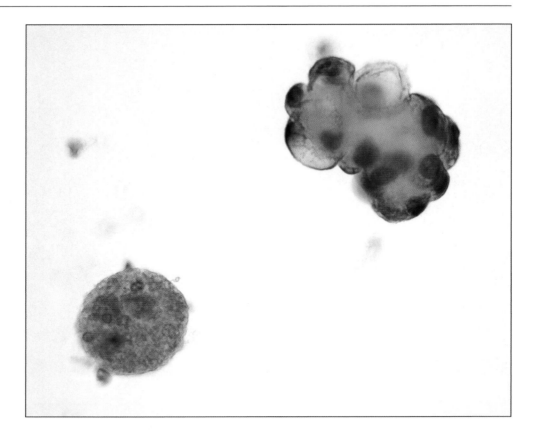

Figure 13.12. Atypical papillary group from a ductal lavage specimen. Note the well-preserved fibrovascular core in the center of the group.

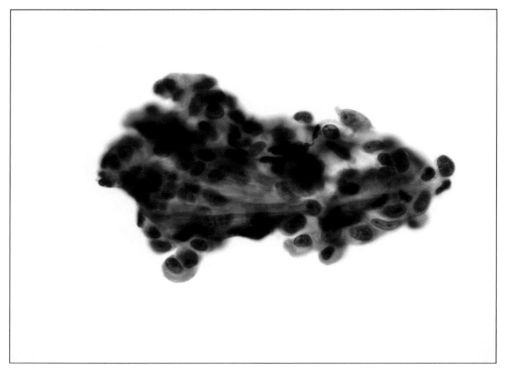

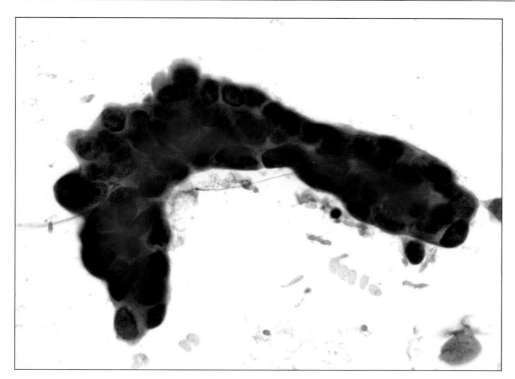

Figure 13.13. Micropapillary carcinoma. The papillary group is composed of very large, irregular nuclei (compare with size of red blood cells) with high nuclear cytoplasmic ratio.

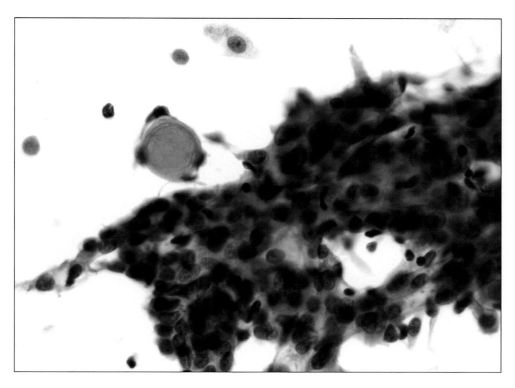

Figure 13.14. Proliferative breast lesion (usual ductal hyperplasia associated with collagenous spherulosis). This smear shows small ductal epithelial cells in a group with associated myoepithelial cells and round structures containing amorphous material.

cellular distribution and components, cell size, and nuclear features can guide the way to define features that may indicate abnormalities to be followed up by excision.

Many benign proliferative lesions can give rise to cellular smears, such as usual ductal hyperplasia in the setting of fibrocystic changes,

Figure 13.15. Proliferative breast lesion (gynecomastia). This smear shows cellular groups composed of tightly cohesive ductal epithelial cells with smooth nuclear contours and associated myoepithelial cells. The florid phase of gynecomastia can produce cellular specimens.

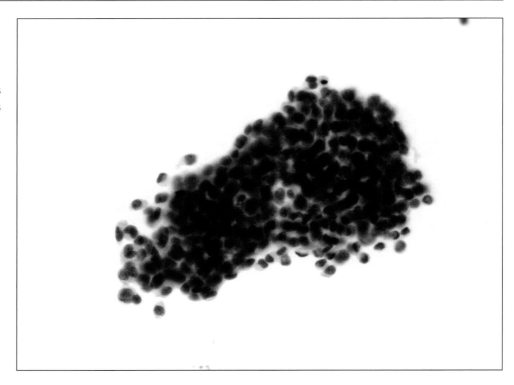

Figure 13.16. Amorphous debris (A) in a scantly cellular smear with few atypical cells (B) from a clinically indeterminate breast lesion. Excision resulted in a histologic diagnosis of ductal carcinoma in situ with comedo-necrosis.

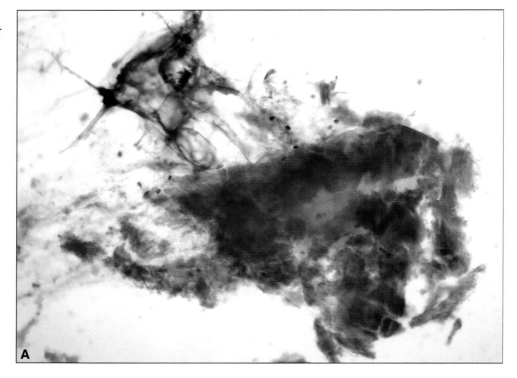

PASH, radial scar, hamartoma, fibroadenoma or, in a male, gynecomastia. Poorly preserved or unintentionally air-dried cytology preparations may alter the morphology in such a way that benign cells appear abnormal.

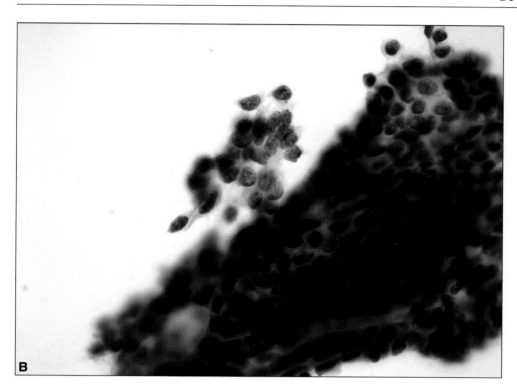

Figure 13.16. *(continued)*

On the other hand, well-differentiated adenocarcinomas or tubular carcinomas may show few, if any single tumor cells, and nuclear hyperchromasia or irregularities can be subtle; the comparison with adjacent groups is often necessary to identify an abnormal population (Figures 13.17 and 18). One has to exercise much caution in interpreting scant smears with few (but abnormal) cells as this may lead to a false-negative report.

CARCINOMA

The most frequent type (approximately 80 percent) of invasive mammary carcinoma is ductal carcinoma. With variations that reflect the range from well- to poorly differentiated tumors and histologic subtypes, the tumor cells occur typically in groups and as single cells. Tumor cells show nuclear atypia, which may include nuclear enlargement, hyperchromasia, increased nuclear-to-cytoplasmic ratio, and irregular nuclear contours. Occasional groups with myoepithelial cells do not exclude ductal carcinoma – it may be difficult to distinguish between ductal carcinoma in situ and invasive ductal carcinoma based on cytologic features, and often ductal carcinoma in situ accompanies invasive carcinoma. The initial clinical management is often similar, so that an exact distinction between ductal carcinoma in situ and invasive carcinoma can be deferred to histologic examination (Figures 13.19–22).

Lobular carcinoma is characterized by small dyshesive tumor cells, mostly in a dense fibrous stroma. Those cytologic samples from may be surprisingly

Figure 13.17. Proliferative breast lesion with atypia. This cytology specimen shows benign ductal epithelial cells (left) and few groups of "atypical" crowded ductal cells (right). Excision resulted in a well-differentiated ductal carcinoma. Due to their tendency to be cohesive and show low nuclear pleomorphism, well-differentiated carcinomas may mimic benign epithelial cells.

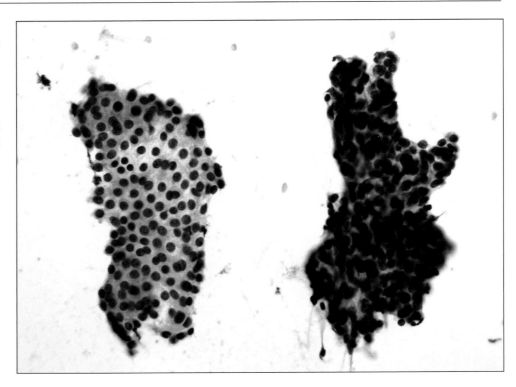

Figure 13.18. A group of "atypical ductal cells" (right side of panel) is present next to benign-appearing ductal cells (SurePath® specimen). A well-differentiated ductal carcinoma was identified on excision.

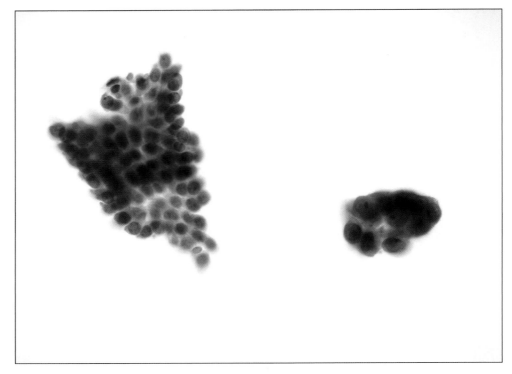

paucicellular – considering the often large breast tumors – and the small tumor cells of classic lobular carcinoma may appear inconspicuous. The cytologic features seen on high-power views are subtle, such as intracytoplasmic vacuoles, inspissated mucin droplets ("targetoid cells"), and signet-ring morphology (Figure 13.23).

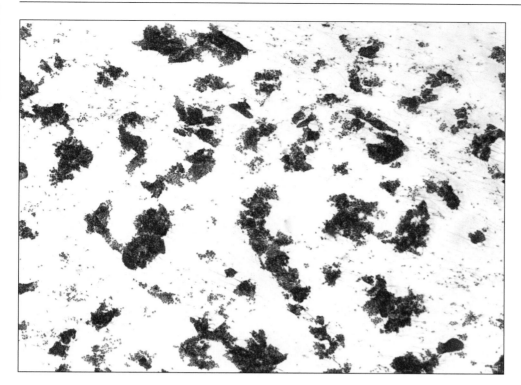

Figure 13.19. Ductal carcinoma. This low-power view shows a markedly hypercellular smear with tumor cells in moderately cohesive groups and singly.

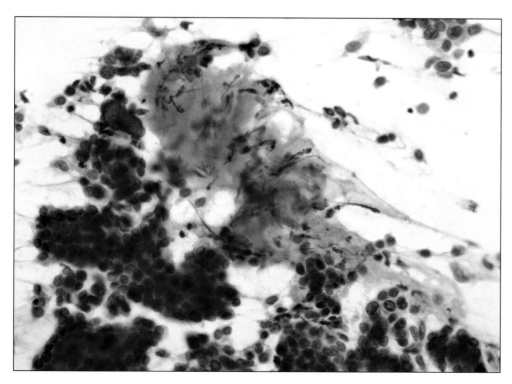

Figure 13.20. Ductal carcinoma. A stromal fragment suggests invasive carcinoma.

Figure 13.21. Ductal carcinoma. The tumor cells are moderately pleomorphic, with irregular hyperchromatic nuclei and increased nuclear cytoplasmic ratio.

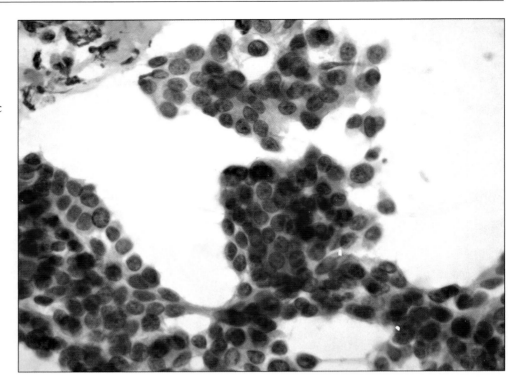

Figure 13.22. Ductal carcinoma, high grade. The tumor cells nuclei are large and markedly pleomorphic with a high nuclear cytoplasmic ratio.

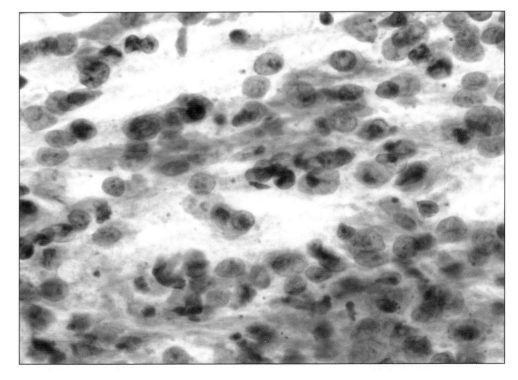

To distinguish invasive lobular carcinoma from lobular neoplasia (lobular carcinoma in situ or LCIS) based on cytology is a challenge, if not impossible (Figure 13.24). The clinical management of invasive lobular carcinoma and lobular neoplasia is different, and cytologic diagnosis should be conservative.

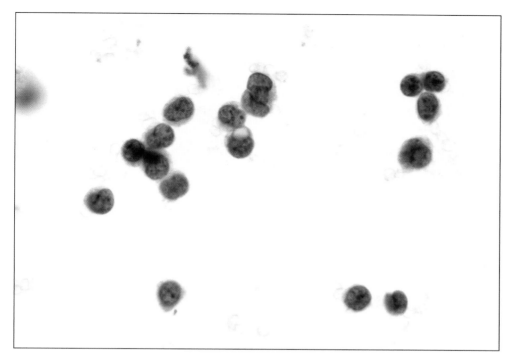

Figure 13.23. Lobular carcinoma. The smear shows dispersed, small tumor cells with slightly irregular nuclear contours and occasional cytoplasmic vacuoles. Excision of this breast mass showed invasive carcinoma, and a negative E-cadherin stain confirmed the lobular subtype.

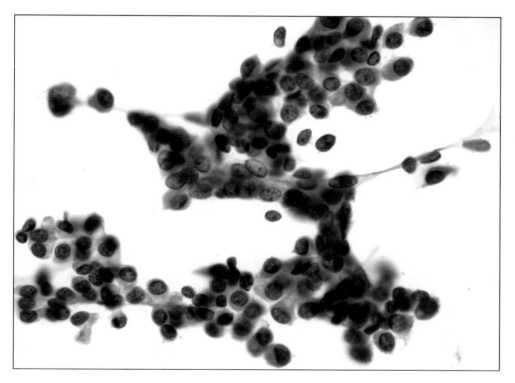

Figure 13.24. Lobular neoplasia. Loosely cohesive groups of cells with lobular morphology are shown. Wide excision of the lesion did not demonstrate invasive carcinoma but extensive lobular carcinoma in situ.

There are many special types of mammary carcinoma, and not all can be discussed here in detail. Special types may include mucinous carcinoma (Figure 13.25), tubular carcinoma, papillary and micropapillary carcinoma, and carcinoma with apocrine or neuroendocrine features. Adenoid cystic carcinoma of the breast is

Figure 13.25. Mucinous (colloid) carcinoma. The invasive tumor cells are present in cohesive groups and appear suspended in abundant background mucin.

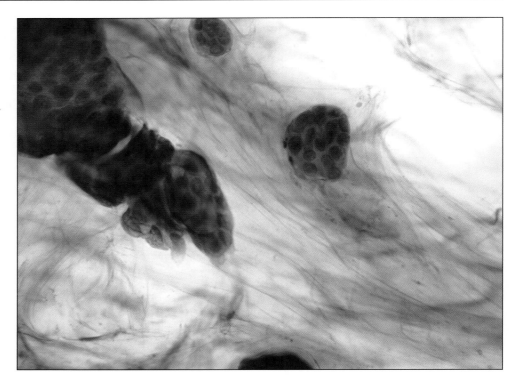

morphologically similar to its counterpart in the salivary gland. Medullary carcinoma of the breast is characterized by high-grade nuclear morphology, a dense lymphocytic infiltrate, and pushing borders – features that require architectural assessment after excision.

METAPLASTIC, MESENCHYMAL, AND SPINDLE CELL LESIONS

Metaplastic carcinomas are a heterogenous group of mammary carcinomas with variable amounts of sarcomatous, spindle cell, or squamoid components (Figures 13.26 and 13.27). Purely mesenchymal tumors of the breast are exceedingly rare. Most malignant breast tumors with a predominantly spindle-cell appearance are either spindle cell carcinomas or phyllodes tumors. For a cytology sample of a breast mass that shows predominantly spindle cells with low nuclear grade, the differential diagnosis may span a wide range from spindle cell carcinoma, phyllodes tumor to fibromatosis (Figure 13.28).

NEWER TECHNOLOGIES

Hormone Receptor and HER-2 Studies in Breast Cancer Diagnostics

Ancillary testing is very important to determine treatment strategies in the multidisciplinary approach to breast cancer. Immunostains for estrogen- and progesterone-receptor proteins, and HER-2 overexpression as well as fluorescent in situ

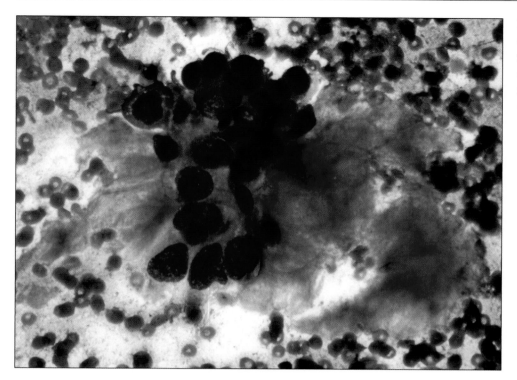

Figure 13.26. Metaplastic carcinoma with chondroid matrix. Tumor cells are embedded in metachromatic, magenta-red matrix material (Giemsa stain).

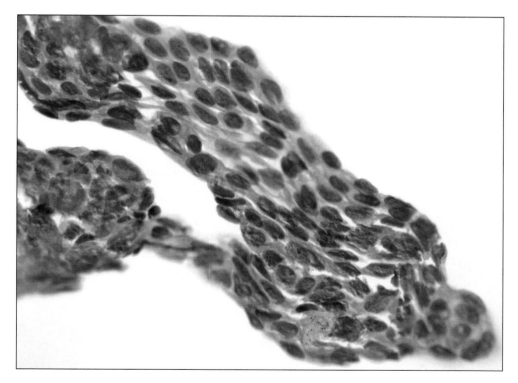

Figure 13.27. Carcinoma with squamoid and spindle-cell features. A flat sheet of tumor cells shows focally spindled cells with well-defined cell borders.

hybridization to test for HER-2 gene amplification can be performed on cytologic material (Figures 13.29 and 13.30). Those tests have to be performed in a standardized setting, and insufficient sampling may present a limiting factor for the evaluation of cytologic preparations.

Figure 13.28. Fibromatosis of the breast. The spindle cells have bland-appearing nuclei and show a wavy pattern.

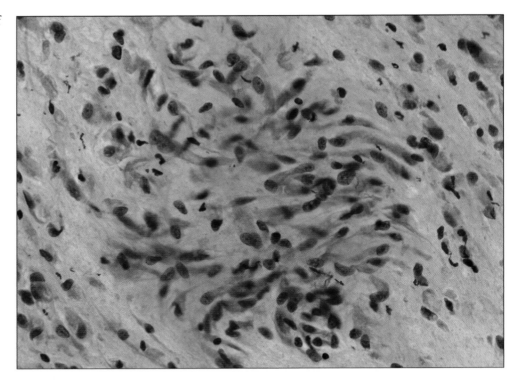

Figure 13.29. Estrogen receptor-positive ductal carcinoma. The positive cells show nuclear staining. Immunoperoxidase stains performed on a smear fixed in 95 percent ethanol (A) and of formalin-fixed cell block (B) show nuclear staining.

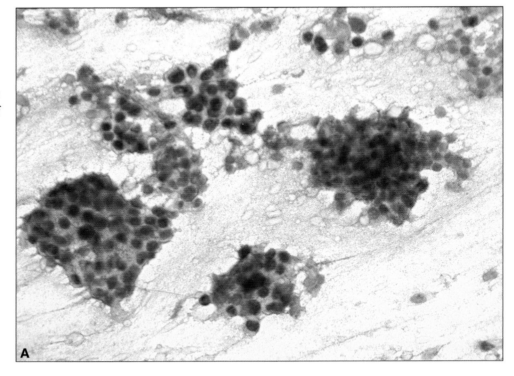

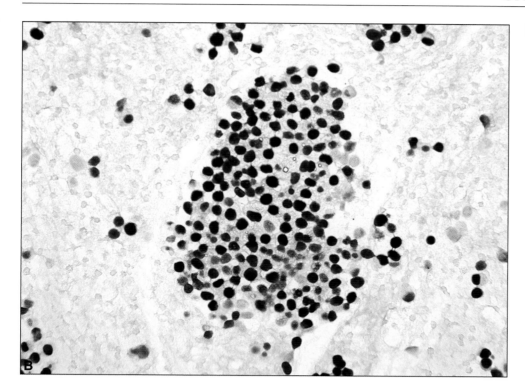

Figure 13.29. *(continued)*

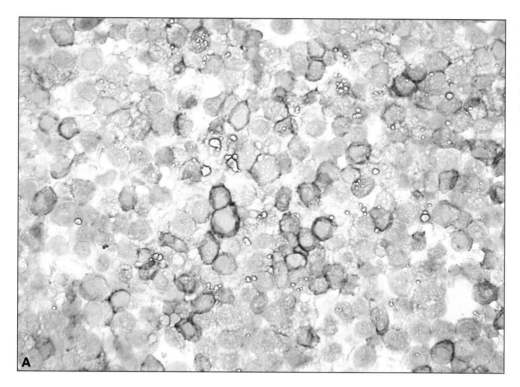

Figure 13.30. HER-2 studies on cell block material. HER-2 immunoperoxidase stain (A) shows some cells with circular staining, interpreted as moderate (2+) overexpression.

Figure 13.30. *(continued)* HER-2 FISH (B) shows red signals labeling the HER-2 gene (not amplified), and the green signals the centromere on chromosome 17. The signals are usually counted for sixty cells and a HER-2/ chromosome 17 signal ratio > 2 would indicate HER-2 amplification.

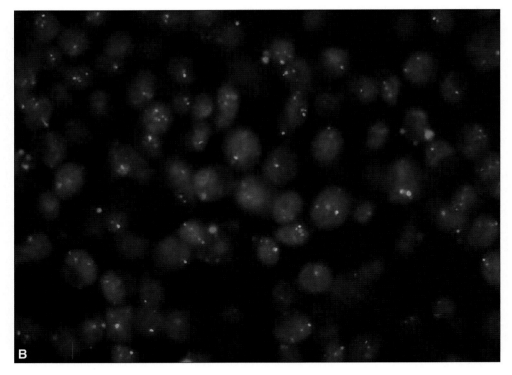

Ductal Lavage Cytology and Nipple Fluid Analysis

Newer, minimally invasive sampling techniques of the mammary duct system are being tested to monitor patients at high risk for breast cancer. These techniques include analysis of spontaneously discharged nipple fluid, ductal lavage which utilizes cannulation of ducts through the nipple, or random periareolar fine needle aspiration. The cytologic findings in those samples are reported in probabilistic categories – benign cells, mild atypia, marked atypia, malignant, or insufficient material for diagnosis (Figure 13.31).

Studies show variable results for cytologic detection of cancerous or precancerous lesions in the breast by duct fluid analysis. The widespread use of ductal lavage as a screening tool has so far been hampered by technical issues and the relatively low sensitivity. At present, random sampling techniques are mostly used in the setting of research and clinical trials. Molecular markers may be employed on duct fluid specimens in the future to better monitor breast cancer risk in individual women.

USE OF IMPRINT CYTOLOGY (TOUCH PREP) IN INTRAOPERATIVE CONSULTATION: MARGIN ASSESSMENT AND SENTINEL NODE EVALUATION

Imprint cytology or touch preparations of surgical specimen use the cells that adhere to a glass slide after gently touching the tissue (Figure 13.32). In contrast to frozen sections, the tissue is left intact for subsequent histologic evaluation. This

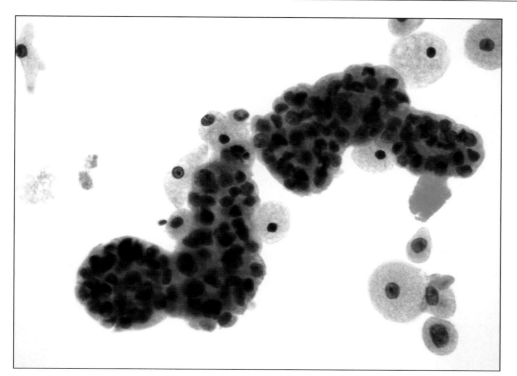

Figure 13.31. Ductal lavage specimen shows groups of ductal cells and histiocytes (mildly atypical).

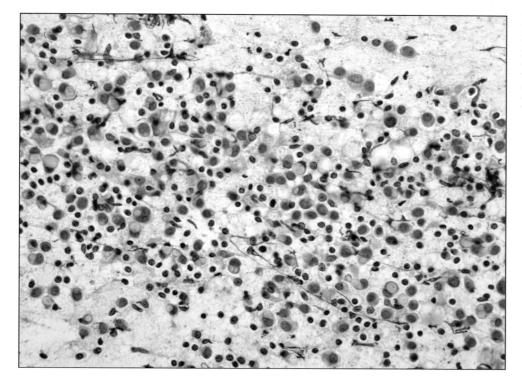

Figure 13.32. Touch prep of metastatic lobular carcinoma in axillary lymph node. The lobular tumor cells are dispersed among small lymphocytes.

approach is particularly useful for rapid/intraoperative interpretation of tissue specimens. Several studies show a sensitivity and specificity profile comparable to frozen sections, with additional applications for rapid interpretation when frozen section is not usually done (for example on core biopsies and for intraoperative margin evaluation). The individual practice of imprint cytology is influenced by clinical scenario, institutional preference, and experience.

Margin evaluation on breast excisions is deferred to permanent sections in most institutions. This is due to the frequent freezing artifacts in breast tissue, and the loss of tissue and morphologic details through freezing. However, margins of surgical excision specimens may be intraoperatively assessed by touch prep without cutting into the tissue.

The same advantage of imprint cytology applies to rapid interpretation of sentinel lymph nodes: touch preps allow rapid sentinel lymph node analysis without necessarily freezing the tissue. This is a method that offers a high specificity in experienced hands with a slightly lower sensitivity for the detection of micrometastases.

REFERENCES

Alkuwari, E. and M. Auger (2008). "Accuracy of fine-needle aspiration cytology of axillary lymph nodes in breast cancer patients: a study of 115 cases with cytologic-histologic correlation." *Cancer* 114(2): 89–93.

Ariga, R., K. Bloom, et al. (2002). "Fine-needle aspiration of clinically suspicious palpable breast masses with histopathologic correlation." *Am J Surg* 184(5): 410–13.

Arun, B., V. Valero, et al. (2007). "Comparison of ductal lavage and random periareolar fine needle aspiration as tissue acquisition methods in early breast cancer prevention trials." *Clin Cancer Res* 13(16): 4943–8.

Ayata, G., G.M. Abu-Jawdeh, et al. (2003). "Accuracy and consistency in application of a probabilistic approach to reporting breast fine needle aspiration." *Acta Cytol* 47(6): 973–8.

Badve, S. S., F. L. Baehner, et al. (2008). "Estrogen- and progesterone-receptor status in ECOG 2197: comparison of immunohistochemistry by local and central laboratories and quantitative reverse transcription polymerase chain reaction by central laboratory." *J Clin Oncol* 26(15): 2473–81.

Bakhshandeh, M., S. O. Tutuncuoglu, et al. (2007). "Use of imprint cytology for assessment of surgical margins in lumpectomy specimens of breast cancer patients." *Diagn Cytopathol* 35(10): 656–9.

Bayramoglu, H., O. Zekioglu, et al. (2002). "Fine-needle aspiration biopsy of invasive micropapillary carcinoma of the breast: a report of five cases." *Diagn Cytopathol* 27(4): 214–17.

Bedard, Y. C. and A. F. Pollett (1999). "Breast fine-needle aspiration. A comparison of ThinPrep and conventional smears." *Am J Clin Pathol* 111(4): 523–7.

Benoit, J. L., R. Kara, et al. (1992). "Fibroadenoma of the breast: diagnostic pitfalls of fine-needle aspiration." *Diagn Cytopathol* 8(6): 643–7; *discussion* 647–8.

Biscotti, C. V., J. H. Shorie, et al. (1999). "ThinPrep vs. conventional smear cytologic preparations in analyzing fine-needle aspiration specimens from palpable breast masses." *Diagn Cytopathol* 21(2): 137–41.

Boerner, S. and N. Sneige (1998). "Specimen adequacy and false-negative diagnosis rate in fine-needle aspirates of palpable breast masses." *Cancer* 84(6): 344–8.

Bofin, A. M., S. Lydersen, et al. (2004). "Cytological criteria for the diagnosis of intraductal hyperplasia, ductal carcinoma in situ, and invasive carcinoma of the breast." *Diagn Cytopathol* 31(4): 207–15.

Brogi, E., M. J. Miller, et al. (2005). "Paired ductal lavage and fine-needle aspiration specimens from patients with breast carcinoma." *Diagn Cytopathol* 33(6): 370–5.

Cangiarella, J., J. Waisman, et al. (2001). "Cytologic features of tubular adenocarcinoma of the breast by aspiration biopsy." *Diagn Cytopathol* 25(5): 311–15.

Chhieng, D. C., J. F. Cangiarella, et al. (1999). "Fine-needle aspiration cytology of spindle cell lesions of the breast." *Cancer* 87(6): 359–71.

Creager, A. J., K. R. Geisinger, et al. (2002). "Intraoperative evaluation of sentinel lymph nodes for metastatic breast carcinoma by imprint cytology." *Mod Pathol* 15(11): 1140–7.

Dawson, A. E. and D. K. Mulford (1994). "Benign versus malignant papillary neoplasms of the breast. Diagnostic clues in fine needle aspiration cytology." *Acta Cytol* 38(1): 23–8.

Dawson, A. E. and D. K. Mulford (1998). "Fine needle aspiration of mucinous (colloid) breast carcinoma. Nuclear grading and mammographic and cytologic findings." *Acta Cytol* 42(3): 668–72.

Dooley, W. C., B. M. Ljung, et al. (2001). "Ductal lavage for detection of cellular atypia in women at high risk for breast cancer." *J Natl Cancer Inst* 93(21): 1624–32.

Fackler, M. J., K. Malone, et al. (2006). "Quantitative multiplex methylation-specific PCR analysis doubles detection of tumor cells in breast ductal fluid." *Clin Cancer Res* 12(11 Pt 1): 3306–10.

Field, A. and A. Mak (2007). "A prospective study of the diagnostic accuracy of cytological criteria in the FNAB diagnosis of breast papillomas." *Diagn Cytopathol* 35(8): 465–75.

Florentine, B. D., B. Staymates, et al. (2006). "The reliability of fine-needle aspiration biopsy as the initial diagnostic procedure for palpable masses: a 4-year experience of 730 patients from a community hospital-based outpatient aspiration biopsy clinic." *Cancer* 107(2): 406–16.

Forbes, R. C., C. Pitchford, et al. (2005). "Selective use of intraoperative touch prep analysis of sentinel nodes in breast cancer." *Am Surg* 71(11): 955–60; *discussion* 961–2.

Frost, A. R., S. O. Tabbara, et al.et al. (2000). "Cytologic features of proliferative breast disease: a study designed to minimize sampling error." *Cancer* 90(1): 33–40.

Fulciniti, F., G. Mansueto, et al. (2005). "Metaplastic breast carcinoma on fine-needle cytology samples: a report of three cases." *Diagn Cytopathol* 33(3): 205–9.

Gornstein, B., T. Jacobs, et al. (2004). "Interobserver agreement of a probabilistic approach to reporting breast fine-needle aspirations on ThinPrep." *Diagn Cytopathol* 30(6): 389–95.

Hermansen, C., H. Skovgaard Poulsen, et al. (1987). "Diagnostic reliability of combined physical examination, mammography, and fine-needle puncture ("triple-test") in breast tumors. A prospective study." *Cancer* 60(8): 1866–71.

Khan, S. A., E. L. Wiley, et al. (2004). "Ductal lavage findings in women with known breast cancer undergoing mastectomy." *J Natl Cancer Inst* 96(20): 1510–17.

Klimberg, V. S., K. C. Westbrook, et al. (1998). "Use of touch preps for diagnosis and evaluation of surgical margins in breast cancer." *Ann Surg Oncol* 5(3): 220–6.

Koss, L. G. (2006). The breast. Koss' diagnostic cytology. L. G. Koss and M. R. Melamed. Philadelphia, Lippincott, Williams & Wilkins. 2.

Lacquement, M. A., D. Mitchell, et al. (1999). "Positive predictive value of the Breast Imaging Reporting and Data System." *J Am Coll Surg* 189(1): 34–40.

Lau, S. K., G. T. McKee, et al. (2004). "The negative predicative value of breast fine-needle aspiration biopsy: the Massachusetts General Hospital experience." *Breast J* 10(6): 487–91.

Lee, A., S. Krishnamurthy, et al. (2002). "Intraoperative touch imprint of sentinel lymph nodes in breast carcinoma patients." *Cancer* 96(4): 225–31.

Levine, P. H., D. Nimeh, et al. (2005). "Aspiration biopsy of nodular pseudoangiomatous stromal hyperplasia of the breast: clinicopathologic correlates in 10 cases." *Diagn Cytopathol* 32(6): 345–50.

Lui, P. C., G. M. Tse, et al. (2007). "Fine-needle aspiration cytology of metaplastic carcinoma of the breast." *J Clin Pathol* 60(5): 529–33.

Mak, A. and A. S. Field (2006). "Positive predictive value of the breast FNAB diagnoses of epithelial hyperplasia with atypia, papilloma, and radial scar." *Diagn Cytopathol* 34(12): 818–23.

Masood, S. (2005). "Core needle biopsy versus fine needle aspiration biopsy: are there similar sampling and diagnostic issues?" *Clin Lab Med* 25(4): vi, 679–88.

Masood, S., A. Loya, et al. (2003). "Is core needle biopsy superior to fine-needle aspiration biopsy in the diagnosis of papillary breast lesions?" *Diagn Cytopathol* 28(6): 329–34.

McKee, G. T. (2002). *Cytopathology of the breast.* New York, Oxford University Press.

McKee, G. T., G. Tildsley, et al. (1999). "Cytologic diagnosis and grading of ductal carcinoma in situ." *Cancer* 87(4): 203–9.

Michael, C. W. and B. Buschmann (2002). "Can true papillary neoplasms of breast and their mimickers be accurately classified by cytology?" *Cancer* 96(2): 92–100.

Myers, T. and H. H. Wang (2000). "Fibroadenoma mimicking papillary carcinoma on ThinPrep of fine-needle aspiration of the breast." *Arch Pathol Lab Med* 124(11): 1667–9.

National Cancer Institute, C. (1997). "The uniform approach to breast fine-needle aspiration biopsy." *Diagn Cytopathol* 16: 295–311.

Ng, W. K. (2002). "Fine needle aspiration cytology of fibroadenoma with multinucleated stromal giant cells. A review of cases in a six-year period." *Acta Cytol* 46(3): 535–9.

Perez-Reyes, N., D. K. Mulford, et al. (1994). "Breast fine-needle aspiration. A comparison of thin-layer and conventional preparation." *Am J Clin Pathol* 102(3): 349–53.

Racz, M. M., R. F. Pommier, et al. (2007). "Fine-needle aspiration cytology of medullary breast carcinoma: report of two cases and review of the literature with emphasis on differential diagnosis." *Diagn Cytopathol* 35(6): 313–18.

Robinson, I. A., G. McKee, et al. (1995). "Lobular carcinoma of the breast: cytological features supporting the diagnosis of lobular cancer." *Diagn Cytopathol* 13(3): 196–201.

Rubin, M., K. Horiuchi, et al. (1997). "Use of fine needle aspiration for solid breast lesions is accurate and cost-effective." *Am J Surg* 174(6): 694-6; *discussion* 697–8.

Saad, R. S., A. Kanbour-Shakir, et al. (2006). "Sclerosing papillary lesion of the breast: a diagnostic pitfall for malignancy in fine needle aspiration biopsy." *Diagn Cytopathol* 34(2): 114–18.

Saqi, A., C. L. Mercado, et al. (2004). "Adenoid cystic carcinoma of the breast diagnosed by fine-needle aspiration." *Diagn Cytopathol* 30(4): 271–4.

Scolyer, R. A., P. R. McKenzie, et al. (2001). "Can phyllodes tumours of the breast be distinguished from fibroadenomas using fine needle aspiration cytology?" *Pathology* 33(4): 437–43.

Sidawy, M. K., M. H. Stoler, et al. (1998). "Interobserver variability in the classification of proliferative breast lesions by fine-needle aspiration: results of the Papanicolaou Society of Cytopathology Study." *Diagn Cytopathol* 18(2): 150–65.

Siddiqui, M. T., M. F. Zakowski, et al. (2002). "Breast masses in males: multi-institutional experience on fine-needle aspiration." *Diagn Cytopathol* 26(2): 87–91.

Simsir, A., J. Waisman, et al. (2001). "Fibroadenomas with atypia: causes of under- and overdiagnosis by aspiration biopsy." *Diagn Cytopathol* 25(5): 278–84.

Simsir, A., J. Waisman, et al. (2003). "Mammary lesions diagnosed as "papillary" by aspiration biopsy: 70 cases with follow-up." *Cancer* 99(3): 156–65.

Sneige, N. (1993). "Fine-needle aspiration of the breast: a review of 1,995 cases with emphasis on diagnostic pitfalls." *Diagn Cytopathol* 9(1): 106–12.

Sneige, N. (2004). "Utility of cytologic specimens in the evaluation of prognostic and predictive factors of breast cancer: current issues and future directions." *Diagn Cytopathol* 30(3): 158–65.

Sneige, N. and G. A. Staerkel (1994). "Fine-needle aspiration cytology of ductal hyperplasia with and without atypia and ductal carcinoma in situ." *Hum Pathol* 25(5): 485–92.

Sneige, N. and A. Tulbah (2000). "Accuracy of cytologic diagnoses made from touch imprints of image-guided needle biopsy specimens of nonpalpable breast abnormalities." *Diagn Cytopathol* 23(1): 29–34.

Subcommittees, N. C. I. F.-N. A. o. B. W. (1997). "The uniform approach to breast fine-needle aspiration biopsy." *Diagn Cytopathol* 16(4): 295–311.

Tafjord, S., P. J. Bohler, et al. (2002). "Estrogen and progesterone hormone receptor status in breast carcinoma: comparison of immunocytochemistry and immunohistochemistry." *Diagn Cytopathol* 26(3): 137–41.

Tavassoli, F. A. and P. Devilee (2003). *Tumours of the breast. Tumours of the breast and female genital organs.* Lyon, IARC Press.

Thomas, P. A., J. Cangiarella, et al. (1995). "Fine needle aspiration biopsy of proliferative breast disease." *Mod Pathol* 8(2): 130–6.

Tse, G. M. and T. K. Ma (2000). "Fine-needle aspiration cytology of breast carcinoma with endocrine differentiation." *Cancer* 90(5): 286–91.

Tse, G. M., T. K. Ma, et al. (2008). "Fine needle aspiration cytology of papillary lesions of the breast: how accurate is the diagnosis?" *J Clin Pathol* 61(8): 945–9.

Ustun, M., A. Berner, et al. (2002). "Fine-needle aspiration cytology of lobular carcinoma in situ." *Diagn Cytopathol* 27(1): 22–6.

Valdes, E. K., S. K. Boolbol, et al. (2007). "Intra-operative touch preparation cytology; does it have a role in re-excision lumpectomy?" *Ann Surg Oncol* 14(3): 1045–50.

Vetto, J. T., R. F. Pommier, et al. (2005). "Breast fine-needle aspirates with scant cellularity are clinically useful." *Am J Surg* 189(5): 621-5; *discussion* 625–6.

Vladescu, T., J. Klijanienko, et al. (2004). "Fine-needle sampling in malignant phyllodes tumors: clinicopathologic study of 22 cases seen at the Institut Curie." *Diagn Cytopathol* 31(2): 71–6.

Wang, H. H., B. S. Ducatman, et al. (1989). "Comparative features of ductal carcinoma in situ and infiltrating ductal carcinoma of the breast on fine-needle aspiration biopsy." *Am J Clin Pathol* 92(6): 736–40.

Wolff, A. C., M. E. Hammond, et al. (2007). "American Society of Clinical Oncology/College of American Pathologists guideline recommendations for human epidermal growth factor receptor 2 testing in breast cancer." *J Clin Oncol* 25(1): 118–45.

INDEX

ACC. *See* adenoid cystic carcinoma, 153, 172–174, 229
adenoid cystic carcinoma (ACC), 153, 172–174, 229
adenomas
    fibrous. *See* fibroadenomas
    nipple adenoma, 57–64, 65
    syringomatous adenoma, 63, 64–65
adenosis, 10–18
    apocrine, 10–11, 174
    microglandular (MGA), 14–18, 150
    nodular, 10
    sclerosing, 10–11, 101, 113, 150, 175
adenosis tumor, 10
adenosquamous carcinoma, 65
ADH. *See* atypical ductal hyperplasia
ALH. *See* lobular neoplasia (LN), noninvasive
anatomy of the breast, 1
angiosarcoma, 205–210
apocrine adenosis, 11, 174
apocrine features, invasive carcinomas with, 174–176
apocrine metaplasia, 2–8, 62
atypia
    proliferative lesions with, 219–225
    radiation-related, 29
atypical ductal hyperplasia (ADH), 122–123
atypical ductal hyperplasia (ADH).
    collagenous spherulosis distinguished, 22
    nipple adenoma distinguished, 64
    papillary lesions and, 70, 75, 76
atypical hemangiomas, 209
atypical lobular hyperplasia (ALH). *See* lobular neoplasia (LN), noninvasive
atypical vascular lesions, 210

basal phenotype, NST carcinomas with, 195
benign stromal lesions, 81–92
BRCA1-related cancers
    basal phenotype, NST carcinomas with, 195
    medullary carcinoma, 159, 162

capillary hemangiomas, 85
carcinoma
    adenosquamous, 65
    DCIS. *See* ductal carcinoma in situ
    encysted or encapsulated papillary carcinoma, 73–75, 77
    fat necrosis obscuring, 29
    intraductal papillary carcinoma, 70–72
    invasive ductal carcinoma, 137, 185
    invasive NST. *See* invasive no special type (NST) carcinomas
    invasive special type. *See* invasive special type carcinomas
    LCIS. *See* lobular neoplasia (LN), noninvasive
    metaplastic. *See* metaplastic carcinoma
    mixed NST and special type, 138
    nipple adenoma distinguished, 64
    radiation atypia and, 29
    spindle cell, 87, 199–203, 230
cavernous hemangiomas, 85
cigarette smoking and duct ectasia, 26
clear cell (glycogen-rich and lipid-rich) carcinomas, 171, 176–177
clear cell metaplasia, 6
CNB. *See* core needle biopsy
collagenous spherulosis, 22, 101, 111
columnar cell change/hyperplasia associated with tubular carcinoma, 148
comedo-type DCIS, 55–57
comedo-type necrosis, LCIS with, 105, 113, 120
complex sclerosing lesions (radial scar), 22, 101, 113, 150
core needle biopsy (CNB)
    fine needle aspirations, replacing, 213
    LN, diagnosis of, 119
    phyllodes tumor, diagnosis of, 52
    special type features, invasive carcinomas with, 138
cribriform carcinoma, invasive, 148, 154, 173
cribriform DCIS, 153
cytology of the breast, 213–236
    cost-effectiveness of, 213
    ductal lavage, 234

fibroepithelial lesions, 218
fine needle aspiration, 234
hormone receptor and HER-2 studies, 232
imprint cytology (touch preparations), 213, 236
invasive carcinomas, 225–230
metaplastic, mesenchymal, and spindle cell lesions, 230
nipple fluid analysis, 234
papillary lesions, 218
preparation of samples, 214–216
proliferative lesions, 219–225
quality of sample, 214
reporting, 214

DCIS. *See* ductal carcinoma in situ
diabetic mastopathy, 30–32
duct ectasia, 27
ductal carcinoma in situ (DCIS), 124–135
ductal carcinoma in situ (DCIS)
    ADH distinguished, 122
    collagenous spherulosis distinguished, 22
    comedo-type DCIS, Paget's disease as form of, 55–58
    encysted or encapsulated papillary carcinoma, management of, 78
    LN, distinguishing, 101, 118
    papillary lesions and, 70, 76
    PLCIS and, 96, 106
ductal carcinoma in situ (DCIS)
    ILC associated with, 142
ductal carcinoma in situ (DCIS)
    tubular carcinoma associated with, 148
ductal carcinoma in situ (DCIS)
    cribriform, 153
ductal carcinoma in situ (DCIS)
    tubulolobular carcinoma associated with, 154
ductal carcinoma in situ (DCIS)
    spindle cell components, 199
ductal carcinoma in situ (DCIS)
    spindle cell components, 201
ductal carcinoma in situ (DCIS)
    cytology of, 225

ductal carcinoma, invasive, 137, 185, 225
ductal hyperplasia, atypical (ADH).. *See* atypical ductal hyperplasia
ductal lavage cytology, 234
ductal neoplasias, 122–135

encysted or encapsulated (intracystic) papillary carcinoma, 73–75, 77, 163
epithelial displacement, 75
erosive papillomatosis (nipple adenoma), 57–65
extensive refraction artifact in invasive NST carcinomas, 168

fasciitis, nodular, 87
fat necrosis, 28–29
fibroadenomas, 37
    hamartomas distinguished, 86
    juvenile fibroadenoma, 42
    LN sometimes involving, 101, 113
    phyllodes tumor distinguished, 51
fibroepithelial lesions, 52, 218
fibromatosis, 87, 89–92
fibrous mastopathy, 31
fine needle aspiration, 213, 234
florid sclerosing duct papillomatosis (nipple adenoma), 234–236
florid usual hyperplasia, 101

glycogen-rich and lipid-rich (clear cell) carcinomas, 171, 176–177
granular cell tumor, 92
granulomatous lobular mastitis, 25
granulomatous mastitis, 25
gynecomastia, 35

hamartomas, 85
hemangiomas, 85, 209
HER-2 studies, 232
histology of the breast, 1
hormone receptor studies, 232
hyperplasia
    ADH. *See* atypical ductal hyperplasia
    atypical lobular (ALH). *See* lobular neoplasia (LN), noninvasive
    florid usual, 101
    pseudoangiomatous stromal (PASH), 81, 210
    tubular carcinoma, columnar cell change/hyperplasia associated with, 148
    usual ductal (UDH), 122–123

idiopathic granulomatous mastitis, 25
IMPC (invasive micropapillary carcinoma), 159, 164–169
imprint cytology (touch preparations), 213, 234–236
inflammation. *See* reactive and inflammatory lesions

intracystic (encysted or encapsulated) papillary carcinoma, 73–75, 77, 163
intraductal papillary carcinoma, 70–72
intraductal papillomas, 67–70, 101, 113
invasive ductal carcinoma, 137, 185, 225
invasive metaplastic carcinoma. *See* metaplastic carcinoma
invasive no special type (NST) carcinomas, 137, 185–186
    ACC differentiated, 173
    extensive refraction artifact, 168
    histology/grading of, 185–186
    IMPC differentiated, 168
    lymphatic invasion by, 168
    metaplastic carcinoma and, 199
    mucinous, 159
    prognostic factors, 187–196
    rare histologic patterns in, 174
    spindle cell components, 199, 201
    with basal phenotype, 195
    with medullary features, 161
    with special type features, 138
invasive special type carcinomas, 137–138
    adenoid cystic (ACC), 153, 172–174, 229
    clear cell (glycogen-rich and lipid-rich), 171, 176–177
    cribriform, 148, 151–154, 173
    cytology of, 225–230
    lobular (ILC), 138–146, 154
    medullary, 159–162, 230
    micropapillary (IMPC), 159–169
    mixed NST and special type, 138
    mucinous, 155–159, 168
    papillary, 162–164
    pleomorphic (PILC), 141, 144
    rare histologic patterns of, 174–179
    secretory, 170–172
    tubololobular, 154–155
    tubular, 65, 151
    with apocrine features, 174
    with neuroendocrine features, 174–179
    with signet-ring cell features, 177

juvenile (secretory) carcinoma, 170
juvenile fibroadenoma, 42

lactation, changes to breast during, 1
LIN (lobular intraepithelial neoplasia), 95
lipid-rich and glycogen-rich (clear cell) carcinomas, 171, 176–177
LN. *See* lobular neoplasia (LN), noninvasive
lobular carcinoma
    ctyology of, 225
    in situ (LCIS). *See* lobular neoplasia (LN), noninvasive
    invasive (ILC), 138–146, 154
    tubololobular carcinoma, 155
lobular hyperplasia, aytypical (ALH). *See* lobular neoplasia (LN), noninvasive

lobular intraepithelial neoplasia (LIN), 95
lobular neoplasia (LN), noninvasive, 95
    clinical features, 96
    comedo-type necrosis, LCIS with, 105, 113, 120
    differential diagnosis, 108–118
    ILC, associated with, 142
    LIN, 95
    microscopic features of, 96–108
    pagetoid involvement of larger ducts, 96
    PLCIS, 95, 96, 106, 113, 120
    treatment and prognosis, 118–120
    tubular carcinoma associated with, 148
    variant forms, 105–106
    with signet-ring cell features, 106
lymphatic invasion by invasive NST carcinomas, 168
lymphocytic mastopathy, 32
lymphoma
    diabetic mastopathy distinguished, 32
    ILC distinguished, 145
    MALT, 32

MALT. *See* mucosa-associated lymphoid tissue lymphoma, 32
mastitis, 25
medullary carcinoma, 159–162, 230
mesenchymal lesions, 230
metaplasias, 2–8
metaplastic carcinoma, 87, 204
    cytology of, 230
    phyllodes tumor distinguished, 52
    spindle cell carcinoma, 87, 203, 230
    squamous cell carcinoma, 203
    with osteochondroid differentiation, 203–204
metastatic lesions
    IMPC differentiated, 168
    papillary carcinoma differentiated, 163
microglandular adenosis (MGA), 14–19, 150
micropapillary carcinoma, invasive (IMPC), 159, 164–170
mucinous carcinoma, 159, 168
mucocele-like lesions, 157
mucosa-associated lymphoid tissue (MALT) lymphoma, 32
myofibroblastomas, 87–89
myoid hamartomas, 85
myoid metaplasia, 7

neuroendocrine features, invasive special type carcinomas with, 178–179
nipple discharge
    cytologic analysis of, 234
    duct ectasia, 25
    nipple adenoma, 58
    papillary lesions, 67
nipple lesions
    nipple adenoma, 57–63, 64, 65
    Paget's disease, 55–57, 58
    syringomatous adenoma, 64–65

no special type (NST) carcinomas, invasive. *See* invasive no special type (NST) carcinomas

nodular adenosis, 10

nodular fasciitis, 87

noninvasive carcinoma. *See* carcinoma

normal anatomy and histology of the breast, 1

NST (no special type) carcinomas, invasive. *See* invasive no special type (NST) carcinomas

osteochondroid differentiation, metaplastic carcinoma with, 203–204

pagetoid involvement of larger ducts in noninvasive LN, 96

Paget's disease of the nipple, 55–57, 58

papillary carcinoma
    encysted or encapsulated, 73–75, 77, 163
    intraductal, 70–72
    invasive, 162–164, 168

papillary lesions, 67–78, 218

papillomas, intraductal, 67–70, 101, 113

papillomatosis, erosive (nipple adenoma), 57–64, 65

PASH. *See* pseudoangiomatous stromal hyperplasia, 81, 210

periductal mastitis, 26

phyllodes tumor, 43–52

PILC. *See* pleomorphic invasive lobular carcinoma, 141, 144

plasma cell mastitis, 25

plasmacytoma, 145

PLCIS. *See* pleomorphic LCIS, 95, 96, 106, 113, 120

pleomorphic invasive lobular carcinoma (PILC), 141, 144

pleomorphic LCIS (PLCIS), 95, 96, 106, 113, 120

proliferative lesions, 219–225

pseudoangiomatous stromal hyperplasia (PASH), 81, 210

radial scar (complex sclerosing lesions), 19–22, 101, 113, 150

radiation atypia, 29

reactive and inflammatory lesions
    diabetic mastopathy, 30–34
    duct ectasia, 27
    fat necrosis, 28–29
    gynecomastia, 35
    mastitis, 25
    radiation atypia, 29

sarcoma, 205–210
    metaplastic carcinoma distinguished, 199
    phyllodes tumor distinguished, 52

sclerosing adenosis, 10–11, 101, 113, 150, 175

sclerosing duct papillomatosis, subareolar (nipple adenoma), 234–236

sclerosing lesions, complex (radial scar), 19–22, 101, 113, 150

sclerosing lymphocytic lobulitis, 31

secretory carcinoma, 170–172

signet-ring cell features
    invasive carcinomas with, 177
    noninvasive LN with, 106

smoking and duct ectasia, 26

solid papillary carcinoma, 70–72

solitary fibrous tumor, 88

spindle cell carcinoma, 87, 199–203, 230

squamous cell carcinoma, 203

squamous differentiation admixed with spindled component, 199, 201

subareolar sclerosing duct papillomatosis (nipple adenoma), 234–236

syringomatous adenoma, 63, 64

terminal ductal-lobular unit (TDLU), 1

breast. *See also* specific conditions, e.g. metaplastic carcinoma
    CNB of. *See* core needle biopsy
    cytology of. *See* cytology of the breast
    histology of, 1
    lactational changes to, 1
    normal anatomy and histology, 1

touch preparations (imprint cytology), 213, 234–236

tubololobular carcinoma, 154–155

tubular carcinoma, 65, 146–151

usual ductal hyperplasia (UDH), 122–123

vascular lesions, atypical, 210